I0490470

Holistic Nursing Home Management in the Era of Change

Holistic Nursing Home Management in the Era of Change

A Pathway To a Sustainable Nursing Home Quality

Joseph A. Umoren

Copyright © 2021 by Joseph A. Umoren.

Library of Congress Control Number: 2021911891
ISBN: Softcover   978-1-6641-7994-3
                   eBook   978-1-6641-7993-6

All rights reserved. No part of this book may be reproduced or transmitted in any form or by any means, electronic or mechanical, including photocopying, recording, or by any information storage and retrieval system, without permission in writing from the copyright owner.

Any people depicted in stock imagery provided by Getty Images are models, and such images are being used for illustrative purposes only. Certain stock imagery © Getty Images.

Print information available on the last page.

Rev. date: 08/27/2021

To order additional copies of this book, contact:
Xlibris
844-714-8691
www.Xlibris.com
Orders@Xlibris.com
828954

Contents

Preface

In nature, all aspects of human life can be likened to a starting sunrise unto sunset, birth unto death, and everything else in between. We value the uniqueness inherent in each stage of the human life cycle, which is characterized either by a state of independence or dependence on others for physiological, economic, psychosocial, and health care needs. Because of the tapestry in human life—failure and success, happiness and unhappiness, pain, sickness, and even death—there is a need for human beings to develop adequate management skills and approaches necessary to solve personal and organizational problems, to provide human needs, and assure societal peace and prosperity. Additionally, it is the interplay that exists between personal, organizational life and the level of social and ethical values of the larger society that has brought our attention to the importance of the holistic management in organizations, especially in nursing homes, as the centerpiece of our ensuing discussion. A nursing home is defined as an institution where people who are old, infirm, and sick live and receive care from others because they are no longer able to care for themselves.

Research studies have shown that our organizational or personal lives can be cyclical, unintegrated, interrupted with misfortunes, and often yearning for a state of wellness, stability, and completeness. The truism is that regardless of our human endeavors in life, such as seeking health and wellness, starting or managing a business, raising a family, getting an education, finding a job, working on a job, or caring for others, the existent tendency for life's fluctuations demands our personal determination and responsibility to be self-reliant to be able to choose alternative courses of action to remain whole. It is only the determinists who would accept that all human behaviors or situations are predetermined, and that there is nothing we can do once they occur. Charles Darwin (1809–1882) postulated a similar argument in his 1859 publication *On the Origin of Species,* and was found to be incompatible with the concepts of human self-determination, human motivation, and holistic management. In holistic management, what we become later in life, personal or organizational, is a product of our decisions and not of predestination.

The human person, as well as human organization, is a system made up of many subparts, which requires the managing, monitoring, and nurturing of all parts so that the entire system is not in a constant state of flux. Inherently, there is nothing abnormal about the seasonality or cyclical nature of human life or human organization regarding its occasional tendency to drift toward disintegration. The abnormality, as we see it, lies on individuals who expect the human life, personal or organizational, to be a smooth ride and therefore fail to be emotionally and spiritually prepared to accept the challenge of seeking its fullness and integration.

It is in this context that Foroux (2020) pointed out in an article, "On the Cyclical Nature of Life," that "the main lesson I learned is that nothing in life is static . . . understanding where we are in a cycle helps us to make better decisions" (Wikipedia 2020, para 10–11). Simwanza (1918), in another article titled "On the Cyclical Nature of Life," stated that "Life can be a maze. As we get older, we have to be less content with only walking the maze. We have to be a little smarter about the way decisions we make and the directions we take" (Wikipedia 2020, para 4).

The important lesson to be learned about the nature of human life is that it demands our constant search for its meaning—a state of completeness and of equilibrium that lies in the concept of holism. It is noteworthy that finding solace, encouragement, and guidance to overcome life's vicissitudes is a virtue that is hidden in our self-determination to persevere, to learn anew, to ask questions, and seek help, knowing that as Plato put it, "Excellence is not a gift, but a skill that takes practice. We do not act rightly because we are excellent, in fact we achieve excellence by acting rightly."

In much the same vein, Fabry (1968, 17) in his book entitled *The Pursuit of Meaning,* pointed out how logo-therapeutic practice applies to real-life struggles, stating: "we do not know our limitations until we try to overcome them—by actions where possible, by attitude where necessary."

In 1996, I wrote an article entitled "Maslow's Hierarchy of Needs and OBRA 1987: Toward Need Satisfaction by Nursing Home Residents." Maslow's hierarchy of needs theory was used to demonstrate the importance of needs satisfaction to human beings in order for them to achieve their psychosocial equilibrium. By using the hierarchy of needs theory as a backdrop to assess needs satisfaction in nursing homes, the article, in part, illustrated the existence of several functional departments within nursing homes, and their expected contributions to each resident's quality of care, quality of life, the environment, and resident fund management.

All managerial, clinical, technical, and expert contributions from each of these nursing home departments were evaluated as essential and were expected to hierarchically and holistically deliver different aspects of residents' needs along Maslow's hierarchy of human needs theory. These ranged from physiological, safety, love and belonging, esteem, and self-actualization needs—in that order.

Implicated also in the hierarchy of needs theory is the order by which human needs must be carefully managed to achieve complete satisfaction before moving onward to avoid psychosocial trauma in humans. However, the article found major misgivings that were not only contradictory to the concept of holistic management but also the presumptive causation for inadequate delivery of nursing home quality. Needing correction is the lack of an integrative and holistic systems approach, which needs different functional departments and stakeholders to see themselves as one holistic team to ensure that residents have their total needs satisfaction from the lower to the higher level needs. By inferences, effective, coordinated decision-making and across-the-board communication were impaired.

Consequently, nursing home residents ended up receiving more of the lower level (basic) needs than their higher level (mega) ones. The critical message about Maslow's needs theory to health-care providers, especially in nursing homes, is that residents' basic needs and mega needs must be satisfied consistently. Basic needs deficiencies do not need extra triggers for them to manifest themselves in humans as they are always in an agitation mood, but mega needs require care providers' assessment and intervention, which otherwise can lead to neglect in care (Umoren, 1996).

Holistic Nursing Home Management in the Era of Change: A Pathway to a Sustainable Nursing Home Quality discusses different topics about nursing homes, emphasizing a holistic approach to management that can be extrapolated to other businesses as well.

Holistic management practice means that all parts of a human organization must be integrally managed as one whole. The approach to holistic management emphasizes the importance of individuals learning to think deeply, see organizational situations broadly, and examine their decision-making processes carefully in order to lower their personal and organizational opportunity costs. In general, holistic management is the reshaping of the traditional management approach in response to the modern-day millennial work-life organizational integration and social inclusiveness. Inclusiveness means no part of the human organization should be ignored or regarded as unimportant. Integration means assigning an absolute value to all parts of the system and managing them equally for the survival of the system as a whole.

The concept of "absolute versus relative" value is important in understanding holistic management. For something to be absolutely valuable, its value has to be independently significant and indispensably related to other parts for the survival of the whole. For example, the human heart has an absolute value in relation to the whole human person for him to survive. Holistic nursing home management is a reminder of an absolute value inherent in each resident's need.

With respect to nursing homes, our intention is multifold: to provide our readers with insights into the evolutions and progress that have occurred within the nursing home industry, from the almshouse/poorhouse to the present-day nursing home management; to help nursing home administrators, managers, and staffers assimilate the fundamentals and framework of change needed to modernize their managerial, supervisory, technical, and clinical functions, not only to understand the resident's holistic needs concept but also to advocate the importance of organizing all parts of their organizations into one whole in order to achieve nursing home quality.

In the aftermath of almshouses and poorhouses, the nursing home industry is perceived by many to be making significant progress in caring for the sick and the elderly. However, to reach its preeminence, recognizing its operational complexities, its uniqueness as a human organization, the importance of "connecting the dots" between all functional parts, must be put into proper perspective. Our hope is to redirect the sizable number of nursing homes still mired in underperformance and cyclical performance toward performance improvement in nursing home quality by using a holistic management approach. In short, care providers in nursing homes will benefit from learning the evolutions and progress in the nursing home industry, past management history, present management approach, and the proposed holistic management approach to help them traverse the future.

It is noteworthy that looking for a single parameter that defines nursing home quality is likely to be unsuccessful. Nursing home quality is a conglomerate of medical, psychosocial, physical, and environmental conditions affecting the health and well-being of each resident. The annual survey reports and the 5-star rating oftentimes interpreted as a measurement of nursing home quality can be misleading. In the end, it is the consistent and daily practice of holistic resident-centered care management and the holistic management of the nursing home operation as a business enterprise that produce a sustainable nursing home quality.

Definition of Terms

We hereby acknowledge that some of the words or phrases listed below may be defined differently or used interchangeably within the text. We are therefore asking our readers for caution: nursing homes, nursing facility, skilled nursing facility, long-term care facility, management, leadership, a manager, a leader, staff, staffer, employee, holistic, comprehensive, entirety, resident, patient, care provider, caregiver.

Delimitation

According to the CBO (Congressional Budget Office) and NHE (National Health Expenditure) data, Medicaid expenditures to nursing homes in the United States was projected to grow by 4 percent from $369 billion to $406 billion in 2019, and expected to increase further beyond 2020. Medicaid remains the primary source of government funding to nursing homes. We have acknowledged the importance of effective financial management and adequate government funding, not only as a part of promoting holistic management but also as what is needed to enhance a day-to-day nursing home business operation.

We do also acknowledge that there is a direct link existing between taxpayers' government funding and their ongoing demand for improved nursing home quality. Therefore, our focal point in this discussion will not include financial management in nursing homes or government funding as a causation for poor nursing home quality. We will be limited to analyzing and providing new ideas and issues beyond government regulations on how to improve poor nursing home quality, what causes it, and how to achieve a sustainable improvement. In doing so, we don't purport to have all answers to all misgivings in nursing homes, but we do believe that embracing a holistic management approach will move the search for nursing home quality in the right direction. Please note that due to the revisions in the nursing facility CFR483 in 2017, both versions are cited in the text (see appendix A).

Acknowledgments

The advancements in the nursing home industry to become a viable healthcare institution as we know it today would not have happened without the vision, steadfastness, conviction, public or private financial support, and social advocacy of countless people, governments, and organizations throughout history. Their basic belief that all human beings from cradle to grave deserve to live with dignity and respect, and receive the best healthcare they need when they are either old, sick, or infirm is enduring. We owe them all a big dose of gratitude and thanks.

Historically, the road of transforming the indignity of almshouses into our modern nursing homes has been long and certainly not easy. The crusade that has been led and continues to be led by many gerontologists, geriatric practitioners, health educators, direct caregivers, regulators, and religious leaders deserves a joining of hands to acknowledge them for their dedication, contributions, advocacy, and support for nursing home reforms on behalf of millions of our citizens who are receiving care in these institutions.

My motivation to write *Holistic Nursing Home Management in the Era of Change: A Pathway to a Sustainable Nursing Home Quality* is to provide an extension of my long career as a licensed nursing home administrator in the United States and advocate for a better management approach that enhances a better quality of life for those who, as a result of life's vicissitudes or normal aging process, are institutionalized in nursing homes. Based on the popular saying "experience is the best teacher," I am therefore propagating holistic management as a better approach to managing human organizations such as nursing homes.

Regardless of any issue affecting the industry that I may have missed, I hope that the experiential and the empirical knowledge this book provides will be helpful in your future management endeavors. I realize that I have arrived where I am now, but not alone. There are many shoulders I stood on. Consequently, I want to thank the following; notably, Mr. Joseph Miller, Ms. Alberta Brasfield, Mr. Saul Bernstein, and others I may have forgotten to mention, for all the professional support and encouragement I received from them as my mentors, supervisors, and friends.

I would also like to thank my wife Deborah Umoren, and my children Uduakabasi Umoren, Imaobong Umoren, and William Harley for their patience and moral support.

Lastly, I want to thank all the health-care workers in nursing homes with whom I had the opportunity to serve. Your dedication and commitment to serve others in need will ever remain invaluable.

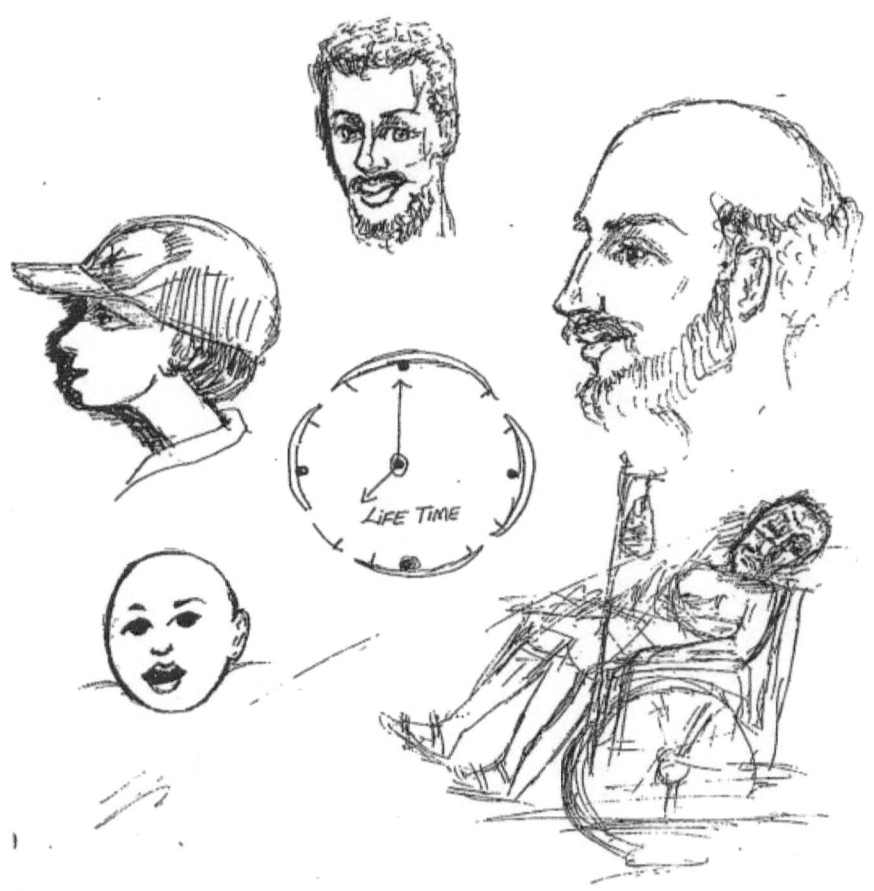

Human Life Stages in the Holistic Health Management Perspective

Chapter 1

Brief History of Management and the Imperative of Holistic Management in Nursing Homes

Before getting deep into the introduction of the concept of holistic management and why it matters in modern-day organizations, let's start with a brief understanding of the history and nature of management as it is practiced today, and how it has evolved over time with new meanings and credibility.

The metamorphosis of management principles has often occurred in response to some emerging new organizational situations, economic circumstances, and human needs that every new generation in management has to face in the pursuit of their organizational goal. Researchers in management principles have estimated the concept of management itself to be relatively new, about 100 to 200 years old, and have also attested to it as being evolutionary and dynamic. For example, during the 1600s and 1700s, none of the early economists like Adams Smith (1723–1790), David Ricardo (1772–1823), and John Stuart Mill (1806–1873) knew or wrote anything about the concept of management. In their views, a national economy depended on the lone interaction of the three factors of production: land, labor, and capital. Additionally, they believed that "economics deals with the behavior of commodities, rather than with the behavior of men" (Drucker, 1973, 21). As classical economists, they also believed in the market economies that were self-regulating in accordance with the natural laws of production and distribution of goods and services.

In colonial America, the concept of management was also unknown. When John Harvard (1607–1638) founded one of oldest Ivy League universities—Harvard University, formally Harvard College—in the United States in 1636, management was not taught, and its business school did not open until 1908. It is generally believed that it is the theory of scientific management by Frederick Winslow Taylor (1856–1915) alongside that of bureaucratic management by Max Weber (1864–1920) that brought the development of management theories to the forefront of American education and on to business practices worldwide.

In 1909, Taylor authored *The Principles of Scientific Management* in support of his idea of management approach. Consequently, the scientific management and bureaucratic management theories—which stressed the philosophy of division of labor, hierarchy of authority, and standardization—were, however, successful in making management the fourth factor of production; namely, land, labor, capital, and management.

Taylorism was criticized for not considering the social needs of workers, pointing only to financial reward in exchange for workers' increased productivity and rejecting the idea that there can be many other ways of doing something, not just one. Scientific management and the bureaucratic management theories are seen to share the same criticisms, especially for creating an impersonal work environment. Nevertheless, some would say that based on those criticisms, new doors were opened to several humanistic management approaches, beginning with the Hawthorne studies in 1924.

The revolution in management theories of the 1950s, 1960s, and 1970s is noted for producing such management theories as systems approach; theory X, Y, and Z; the contingency theory; management by objectives; and total quality management, to name a few.

Contiguous to the concept of scientific management and humanistic management is holistic management. Holistic management is herewith defined as a management concept requiring all organizational members to have the ability for visual and perceptual connections with all of the personal or organizational entities that constitute the whole, especially in decision-making.

The emergence of holistic management can be likened to the New Testament of the Bible in relation to the Old Testament. Just as the purpose of the New Testament is not to abolish the Mosaic laws but to fulfill them or bring it to perfection (Matt. 5:17–18), so is the purpose holistic management in relationship to scientific and humanistic management. The commonality between humanistic and holistic management approaches is noted not only for their advocacy of the importance of employees' productivity, but also the concern for employees' on-the-job well-being. By taking the importance of employees' intrinsic values and their needs satisfaction into consideration, recognizing employees as human capital and asset in any organization, employers are therefore encouraged to embrace expenditures for nurturing and motivating their employees as a smart investment in exchange for increased productivity.

The value of employees in organization is further explained by erasing the long-standing controversy inherent in defining management as science or art. The answer to this controversy is seen as resting on the concept of human capital—the human skills, knowledge, and experience that organizations need to survive, especially in our technological age.

Majority of researchers have seemingly accepted management as both science and art based on standard requirements. As science, the argument for management practice as science is that it is purported to have a cause and effect relationship propelled by human effort, meaning that it is through efficient management that organizational goals are met, and vice versa. As art, management practice is purported to use personal skills of employees that are learned, taught, and updated. It demands continuous learning and hands-on practice based on scientific management theories that are evolutionary, dynamic, and adaptive in time and place. The emergent concept of holistic management not only represents an extension of scientific management and humanistic management, but a management approach that also emphasizes and teaches organizational integration and sound decision-making as the solution to organizational problems. Essentially, today's business managers, as well as future ones, are availed the luxury of utilizing the third management concepts—the holistic management emanating from the scientific and humanistic management approaches—to ensure the much-needed improvement of their business practice, especially in nursing homes, where a significant amount of customer dissatisfaction still abounds.

In a book titled *The Nursing Home Market: Supply and Demand for the Elderly*, Rhoades (1998, 3) saw the necessity to increase quality in nursing homes, and stated that "with increasing life expectancy, an aging population, and the functionally impaired growing, how best to meet long-term care needs continues to challenge policy makers." Accordingly, holistic management is seen as providing the answer by properly identifying two interrelated nursing home components consisting of the direct resident care management beyond the medical/nursing model, and managing nursing homes as a business organization. The two components are symbiotically tied to each other; one component cannot afford to be dysfunctional without adversely affecting the other, nor can we recommend that both components be folded into one.

The frequently cited culprits of poor nursing home care quality is its substandard care by direct caregivers, lack of safety and amenities, to name a few. Even though a holistic management approach is not a new concept in nursing and medicine, it is one that has long been ignored or underutilized in business, clinical, and personnel management practice in nursing homes.

To assure the clarity of purpose and to successfully guide our readers, it is our hope that this presentation will raise the consciousness of nursing home practitioners about the concept of holistic management and its general framework in business management. In nursing homes, the concept of holistic management approach is purported to relate to resident care management, decision-making, resource management, staff supervision, barriers and benefits of adopting holistic management, and defining existing theories that support or do not support a holistic approach to management in nursing homes as well as in other business enterprises. Besides, as in the scientific/classical and humanistic management approach, business schools in colleges and universities must develop curricula to teach holistic management. It is through this medium and classroom teaching that business entrepreneurs, healthcare providers, and staff will be sufficiently informed of the benefits of holistic management so as to modify their professional and personal outlook relating to organizational integration and decision-making processes.

Nursing home administrators as leaders will be able to gravitate toward the holistic management approach to become holistic nursing home administrators (HNHAs) in practice, and to join the ranks of other professionals of our time who have already professed holistic management in their practice. Dr. David Allen Brownstein, who is a board-certified "family practitioner and a medical director of the Center for holistic medicine" (Wikipedia 2020, para 1), is our nearest example. Another example is the Holistic Industries, a business enterprise that is not only adopting "holistic" in its business name, but has its mission statement stating, "as our name suggests, we care for the whole person" (Wikipedia, 2020 para 2).

When Aristotle (385–332 BC) wrote his concept of "proportional equality," it implied a holistic and equal treatment of all human persons and groups, as well as all parts of human systems, with resource distribution that is due to them to meet their psychosocial, physical, emotional, and spiritual needs. It is our hope that all organizational leaders, especially in nursing homes, by realizing the meaning of "proportional equality" of parts, will learn to visualize and master all parts of their business operations and their interconnections in order to be able to adequately respond to their operational shortfalls.

In nursing homes, there is a need to provide an adequate response to the multiplicity of nursing home regulations to improve and sustain nursing home quality specific to the needs of residents and staff. To this end, leaders and managers of organizations should practice a daily routine of proactively reviewing and ensuring that different parts of their organization are functionally interconnected, and if not, to determine what needs to be fixed. Such quiet moments taken for an operational reassessment can be rewarding. Proactive operational assessment is consistent with the cliché that "a stich in time saves nine."

The newness and limited exposure of the holistic business management approach compared to the scientific and humanistic management in our current business world should not be a deterrence but a motivator toward the new management approach that is based on sound ancient philosophical principles of holism, as propounded by Florence Nightingale, Hippocrates, and Allan Savory in nursing, medicine, and business practice respectively.

The Hippocratic philosophy in medical practice and that of Florence Nightingale in nursing practice affirmed that in spite of cultural and ethnic variation, disease management, lifestyles changes, and ageing process, managing care delivery in humans is universal and holistic. Ultimately, both Hippocrates (460--70 BC), nicknamed as "the Father of Western Medicine," and Nightingale (1820–1910) also nicknamed "The Lady with the Lamp," saw all human beings holistically, advocating the form of human healing that considers the whole person in the interdependency of the body, mind, and spirit. Nightingale also went on to propound her environmental theory, which described the importance of "nurse's initiative to configure environmental settings appropriate for the gradual restoration of the patient's health, and how external factors associated with the patient's surrounding affect life or biologic and physiologic processes, and his development" (Wikipedia 2017, para. 2).

Nightingale's concept of environmental holism in healthcare settings, especially nursing homes, is not limited to the physical plant. It includes "provision of a quiet or noise-free and warm environment, attending to patient's dietary needs by assessment, documentation of time of food intake, and evaluating its effects on the patient" (Wikipedia 2017, para. 4). She was also concerned about providing pure fresh air, pure water, effective drainage, cleanliness, and light to promote good health and disease management. An article titled "Florence Nightingale and Holistic Philosophy Light" (1997) stated that:

> *Florence Nightingale lived at a time when allopathy and homeopathy were competing for dominance in medical care. Nightingale's philosophy of health and healing was more similar to the holistic philosophy of homeopathy than to the mechanistic philosophy of allopathy. Why, then, did Nightingale align organized Nursing with allopathy medicine? Perhaps Nightingale, always the pragmatist, understood that allopathy would gain the dominant position in medicine. Perhaps aligning nursing with allopathy was a way to ensure the survival and legitimacy of nursing as a profession. Modern*

nursing can reconnect with Nightingale's holistic philosophy by preparing graduates conversant with holistic philosophy and by encouraging research that focusses on how the natural healing process is facilitated (Wikipedia, 2019 para 1).

As care providers in nursing homes, your focus is directed to following care requirements vital to providing a holistic care as advocated by Nightingale. Samuel Hahnemann, a German and founder of homeopathy, more than 250 years ago did not use the phrase *holistic care* but his principle in health care remains the same, that the total treatment of a patient should include his spiritual, emotional, mental, and physical needs.

In much the same vein, Allan Savory (1935–present) introduced holistic management to general business management, calling it "a systems thinking approach to managing resources." However, his early action to prevent the environmental desertification, blaming it on overgrazing by livestock animals and eliminating them, was later considered as myopic in decision-making. Savory's holistic views in managerial decision-making in business and in politics are presumed to stem from the lesson he learned from his earlier decision regarding environmental desertification, confirming that the decisions that we make, personal or organizational, have consequences.

Considering the efficacy of the holistic approach to business management decisions, some researchers have maintained that if Allan Savory had given himself enough time and effort to broaden his thinking (holistically) prior to deciding on culling the elephants, he could have saved both the environment and the livestock. Needless to say, in recent years Allan Savory is regarded as the father of holistic business management. Despite his initial setback in decision-making, Savory's holistic views, particularly on the environmental management, is regarded as having a heuristic value to the current fight against the current global climate change through his atmospheric carbon reduction campaign as well.

By regulation, nursing home administrators and directors of nursing are trained to administratively lead their organizations consistently and holistically to fulfill the OBRA's mandate in providing a "comprehensive care" under the federal, state, and municipal guidelines. In our view, the unfulfilled mandates that still exist despite OBRA '87 do not indicate an insufficiency in government regulations; rather, it tends to represent an insufficiency in not using a holistic management approach in nursing homes.

Care giving in nursing homes requires nursing home management to expand their organizational boundaries, both vertically and horizontally, beyond the narrow, traditional top-down span of control. The epiphany of the holistic management model therefore requires leadership that assures an expansive but integrative, inclusive, and nonlinear approach in nursing home management.

It is the job of nursing home administrators as the facility's leaders to advocate a center-out chain of command in supervision, education, and communication, in which all facets of the nursing home and stakeholders are integrated and coordinated to create a culture of shared interest, responsibility, and accountability. The facility administrator is to determine whether or not his organizational universe and the direct resident care services are comprehensive enough to optimize the organizational and resident-centered care outcomes. It is only when a nursing home administrator is able to discern the complexity of residents' needs, his organization, and imagine himself as a holistic manager standing in the center of his organizational universe will he be able to manage the changing horizon and the regulatory demands in nursing home management.

The essence of holistic management is the ability of a decision maker to perceive the complexity of an organization and to ensure all parts are integrated. Faced with the current negative public opinion of nursing home care, doing something the same way and expecting a different result would fit the definition of insanity. Holistic nursing home management reflects a new approach to managing nursing homes, taking into consideration its organizational and resident care complexity, needing its parts to be integrated as a means of achieving nursing home quality.

The holistic approach to nursing home management is broadly characterized by the belief that all parts of its system are intimately interconnected, explicable only in reference to the whole. The attention of nursing home department directors and staff must be drawn to perceive their departmental services not as separate and unequal in value, but as integrated services directed toward the resident's total care needs. Since

OBRA '87, it is still the unintegrated nursing home services—of which the sum of the parts has not produced the whole—that has brought the risk of the unintended but preventable bad consequences for care recipients, families, and regulators.

It is not in keeping with the holistic health management principles if residents' services are segregated and graded as more important or less important. In holistic health management, nothing can be farther from the truth. In holistic practice, lateness in food delivery or turning and repositioning of residents is as bad as lateness in medication administration. All care services are expected to be delivered adequately and on time. The lack of holistic systems approach in nursing home management can be expressed not only in the inability of a nursing home administrator to see his organization through an extended lens involving integrative stakeholders—staff, residents, families, community, and regulators needing to work together to raise the nursing home quality—but also his inability to empathize with the psychosocial and physical impact on residents of services that are either delayed, insufficient, or not provided.

It is important to remember that for the purpose of regulatory compliance and in the eyes of public opinion, nursing homes services are evaluated as one whole entity, reflecting whether or not the team has lost or gained its cohesiveness of purpose to ensure comprehensive customer satisfaction. It should be remembered that each resident's satisfaction is expressed in terms of the sum total of the quantity and quality of services that are interdisciplinarily 100 percent for the resident's quality of care, quality of life, fund management, and the environment.

Holistic health management in nursing homes recognizes the intricacies and the nature of geriatric caregiving, and requires no stakeholder, internal or external, to be regarded as an independent actor in the pursuit of nursing home quality. Geriatric care involves dealing with residents with fully developed cultural values, religious values, behavior patterns, medical history, psychiatric issues, and perhaps social prejudices.

Because residents' families are in a better position than staff to know the histories and life events of their loved ones, they are strongly encouraged to be consistently involved in caring and rendering constructive advisement to staff. In this case, it is a team effort in which every hand must be on deck to improve nursing home quality and consistently meet regulatory compliance.

For the concept of holistic nursing home management to work, stakeholders referred herein must adopt the attitude of "how can I help" rather than "how can I criticize." The history of nursing homes has always been referred to as "needing improvement" and requiring "new ways of doing things." Historically, it was in 1986 when the nursing home industry was at the lowest point of its existence. A study conducted by the Institute of Medicine (IOM) concluded poor care, ranging from resident abuse, neglect, and insufficient care. The study recommended the Nursing Home Reform Act (NHRA), which became part and parcel of the Omnibus Reconciliation Act of 1987.

The Omnibus Reconciliation Act of 1987 (OBRA '87) was passed by the Congress of the United States of America with specific guidelines aimed at standardizing, improving care and well-being for individuals residing in nursing homes. A close examination of OBRA's document discovers that it also calls for a holistic philosophy of care, designed not only to address every aspect of human needs but to prevent the exclusion of needs deemed by it to be essential for maintaining or improving residents' health and well-being. Essentially, each resident entering a nursing home "must receive and the facility must provide the necessary care and services to attain or maintain the highest practicable physical, mental, and psycho-social well-being in accordance with the comprehensive assessment and plan of care (OBRA, Interpretive Guidelines, 1987, p. 79).

While it is advisable for care providers to master the inherent meaning of the above mandate, it is even more important for them to understand the two platforms in which the word "comprehensive" is implicated. First, there is the clinical platform that requires a comprehensive clinical, psychosocial assessment and treatment of each resident's total needs; and second, there is the management platform requiring not only a full understanding of all parts that constitute the length and breadth of the nursing home, but also how and why all parts should be integrated and managed to form one healthcare and business organization. Understanding these platforms is inherent in understanding the functional relationship between clinical management and personnel management for the planning, organizing, staffing, coordinating, supervising, and controlling necessary to achieve better service outcomes.

Holistic systems approach in nursing home management is designed to help facilities to avoid hit and miss performances still plaguing nursing home quality in most of our nursing homes today. In an article titled "Regulating U.S. Nursing Homes: Are We Learning from Experience?" Walshe (2001) wrote "the quality of care in U.S. nursing homes has been a recurrent matter of public concern and policy attention for more than thirty years . . . the problems of poor quality and neglect and abuse of patients still appear to be endemic" (Wikipedia 2019, para 1).

The OBRA '87 document has approximately 522 F-tags, and is written as a package deal to cover many different aspects of residents' care—sometimes departmentalized as medical, nursing, social services, nutrition, recreation, spiritual/religious, environment, staffing, and recordkeeping; ultimately taken holistically and comprehensively to measure the quality of care, quality of life, fund management, and the environment of individuals residing in nursing homes. Because each F-tag is also known to have multiple parts in regulatory interpretations for possible deficiencies, only those nursing home practitioners with a holistic view of these regulations can be in a better position to avoid deficiencies and poor service. To be holistic would require each care provider, regardless of his station in the nursing home organizational hierarchy, to carefully examine the number of care implications in each of the F-tags to ensure that residents are not receiving partial, substandard care or no care at all.

According to research findings and public opinion, centuries after the concept of almshouses and the poorhouses; over eighty-six years, as of 2021, after governmental financial and regulatory oversight was indicated in the passage of the Medicaid Act of Congress in the United States of America in 1935; and over thirty-four years of OBRA's inception, nursing homes are still considered as having a sizable room for improvement. But it must be pointed out that the uniform standard for measuring NHQ was not posted until 2008, when the Center for Medicare & Medicaid Services (CMS) in the United States worked and achieved its two landmark initiatives; namely, the 5-star rating scale and the MDS (minimum data set) for nursing homes. By using annual surveys and other self-reported quality measures (QM) data on the MDS, CMS is currently able to use three criteria; namely, annual health inspection, quality measures, and nursing staffing to designate high and low performing nursing homes. Even though this improvement is reportedly known to yield dividends in monitoring nursing home quality, it is unclear however why Life Safety survey results is excluded in the CMS star-rating system, given the importance of safety and security in nursing homes. For the purpose of our current presentation, we have determined that in order for the care that each resident receives in a nursing home to be holistic, it is necessary to include, prioritize, and rate the impact the sociophysical environment has on residents to determine the overall nursing home quality. We hope to make this point clearer in the preceding pages of this book.

Practicing nursing home administration demands empathy. There can be no gainsay about the strong emotions that goes into individuals' decision to move from their homes into an institution despite their vicissitudes of life or a diminution in their activity of daily living. Therefore, the initial function of nursing homes is to assure their new admissions that their nursing home placement is a good idea and that their stay will be pleasurable.

In the holistic health management, the importance of a preadmission meeting between the facility's staffers, the resident, and family that is well coordinated, integrated, and transparent cannot be overemphasized. Under Admissions Policy, OBRA '87's interpretive guidelines—CFR483.15 (a) (1), (6), F620 as revised in 2017 and contained in F-Tag Help—stated that "the facility must establish and implement an admissions policy . . . a nursing facility must disclose and provide to a resident or potential resident prior to time of admission, notice of special characteristics or service limitations of the facility" (Wikipedia 2020. para 1, 6). Noteworthy is a difference between the "preadmission meeting" we are advocating and perhaps the PASARR (preadmission screening and resident review) in which one is behavioral, with the goal of establishing a human relationship, and the other clinical, with the goal of establishing the resident's eligibility for admission respectively.

The preadmission meeting between nursing home staffers and nursing home residents with their representatives is deemed meaningful when it is holistic and futuristic in approach, with the goal of establishing and explaining realistic expectations and the vision of creating a partnership between the residents, families, and the facility. Consequently, implicated in residents' post-admission experience are the face validity of staff behavior, the facility's appearance, and keeping the preadmission promises. In nursing homes, it is the controversy of who made the promises, who is delivering on those promises, and what deviations exist that determines the nursing home residency as a curse or blessing for both the resident and the nursing home. Nursing home staffers must be reminded that broken promises lead to mistrust between partners and promises kept lead to trust and friendship between them. Residents who are admitted into nursing facilities are no exceptions. The creation of an atmosphere of trust and partnership between residents, families, and nursing home staffers starts with the preadmission encounters, where everyone usually starts off as total strangers but need to establish a meaningful conversational distance and relationship to survive well.

The psychological resistance of citizens to entering nursing homes has not dissipated. Because families and residents' representatives are still voicing concerns, there tends to be a need to review the management approach in these institutions besides government regulations. Our interest is to advocate for a successful and improved nursing home industry so that citizens can perceive it as their next home in their later years, where caregivers are more efficient in providing their medical, environmental, and psychosocial needs, and are properly recognized and appreciated for the services they provide.

Nursing homes became one of the essential healthcare institutions in our modern societies when our societies progressed from the agrarian to industrial age, meaning "less and less extended families living together and more nuclear families (Mom, Dad, and Kids) and because of this new separation and focus on the individual . . . also families were having fewer kids . . ." (Wikipedia, 2017, para 2).

Because children, grandchildren, nephews, and nieces of the sick and the elderly are no longer homebound, care givers in nursing homes must learn to surrogate by transplanting the traditional family values into their agencies and to provide the best possible care for those individuals who can no longer live on their own.

Being cognizant of the dual nature of the nursing home as the resident's home and as an institution is important. Recognizing that the uniqueness of a nursing home as the resident's home and as an institution that harbors both residents and workers who are not relatives 24/7 has its advantages and disadvantages. Consequently, care givers are mandated to learn how to be professional with the residents to show them compassion, empathy, gentleness, patience, sensitivity, proper demeanor, to name a few.

A typical example of showing respect and protecting the dignity of the residents in their own home is for staffers to knock on the door before entering their rooms in a manner in which we would treat their neighbors in their communities. Staffers are expected to ask them what their needs are instead of playing god for them. These expectations, which are also present in most care manuals, will ensure that the rights of residents as citizens are adhered to from cradle to grave regardless of the health/mental capacity or incapacity of the residents.

The advantages accruing to the residents in nursing homes and their families are noted. Some of the reasons why people are admitted into nursing homes are not limited to the following: their inability to independently care for themselves at home or inability to afford home-based care; the unwillingness or unavailability of an immediate family to do so. In other words, when the individual is no longer considered safe to live in his home unsupervised, safety becomes the overriding reason for nursing home admission. Contrary to the apparent apprehension frequently expressed toward institutionalized care in preference to home-based care, we see both options as plausible under the right circumstances. There is a need for nursing home care to improve to ensure an easier choice and decision-making for residents and families outside some of the reasons we have already asserted for not supporting nursing home placement.

A book titled *Society and Culture* (Merrill, 1969, 276) also emphasized how much our social functions are changing to exclude the functions of the traditional family, which hitherto cared for its sick, infirm, unemployed, and the elderly. Merrill concluded that much of these functions are gone when he wrote that "the family was the one institution to which the individual could look for protection . . . this function has also been taken over in large part by other agencies both public and private." The good news is that like a child at birth, the contemporary nursing home industry is a public utility agency that is slowly outgrowing the syndrome of the almshouse and its negative stereotypes. Nevertheless, it still needs more work, more dedicated care providers with innovative ideas in their management approach involving the residents, community, family, and the government as shareholders. In this vein, we should advocate for more, not less, government support, funding, and regulatory oversight to make nursing homes a home away from home for the residents, affirming the idea that "every society has certain functions that must be performed if it is to survive" (Merrill, 1969, 115).

There is no social responsibility that can be greater than making life better for institutionalized persons in nursing homes. And by embracing holistic nursing home management, it would mean we have entered an era of rationality in nursing home care where piecemeal care and services are declared things of the past.

A	B	C	D	E	F	G
H	I	J	K	L	M	N
O	P	Q	R	S	T	U
V	W	X	Y	Z		

Alphabetical Integration and the Schematic
Concept in Holistic Management

Chapter 2

Meaning and Definition of Holism in Holistic Management Practice

The concept of holism as it applies to human organizations and human persons is worthy of everyone's attention. Empirically it can be understood through having a comprehensive view of what issues impact us individually and organizationally. Human beings are known to operate under a psychosocial and anatomical system of parts requiring integration, coordination, and maintenance. Human organizations have operational systems that require similar attention. It is not uncommon for a system to breakdown because one of its parts has malfunctioned.

To explain the concept of holism and its importance, there are schematic examples and symbols that are already part of our everyday life. In our spoken or written words of the English language culture, we use vowels and alphabets. There are five known vowels and twenty-six letters of the alphabets (A–Z), holistically organized to help humans to learn to formulate sensible words and sentences needed for them to communicate well with one another.

The biblical story of the Tower of Babel is a reminder of what resulted when God (Genesis 11:1–9) confounded the people and disconnected them so they weren't able to communicate with one another. In today's language structure, it means if any of the alphabetical letters is missing in a word's formulation, unintegrated in placement, or unintelligible in meaning, an effective use of human language would be impaired, resulting in confusion.

According to Egyptian mythology (1850–1700 BC), the arrangement of each letter of the alphabet was therefore predesigned to form a perfect union with each other so as to enhance communication when they are constructed for speaking or writing purposes. To ensure the holistic integrity and the importance of the alphabetical structure in the language system, school beginners are often mandated to learn or even memorize all the letters of the alphabet sequentially as a foundation for future learning and communication.

The second example of the schematic meaning of holism in nature is your hand, which is composed of your palm and five fingers. If you have a defective finger that is not functional but still attached, you have a hand but not a whole hand as was designed to perform essential daily functions; meaning that the sum of these parts is not the whole. In this scenario, the whole only exists when all parts in any organized system are functional, healthy, and integrated with other parts.

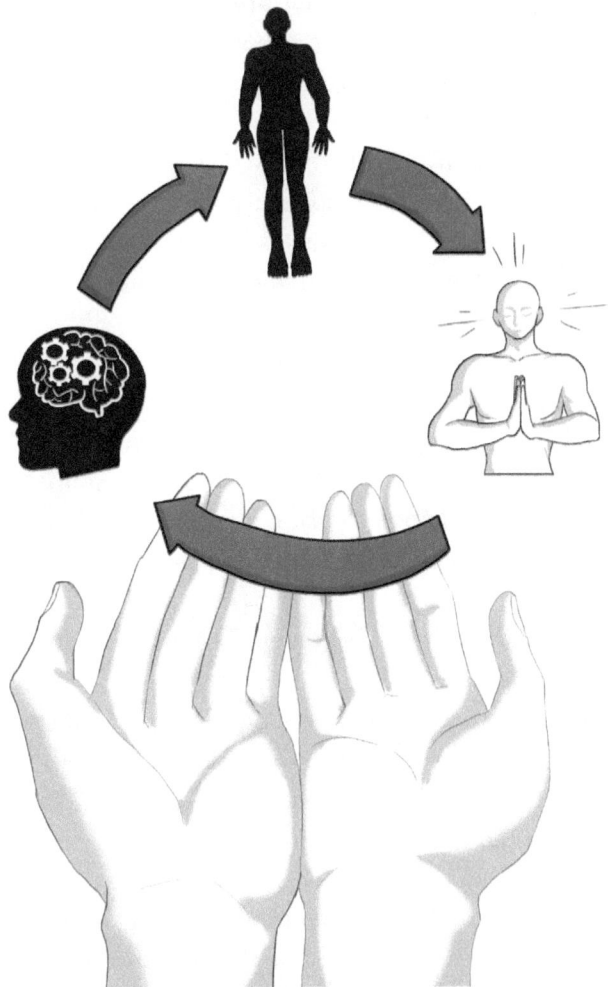

Human Hand with Fingers, Integration and the
Schematic Concept in Holistic Management

The meaning of holism in an organizational setting is the belief that all
assumed and predetermined parts will constitute the whole. The holistic
view of an organization is based on the composite of the functional parts
(departments, clientele, outreaches, and business connections) needed
in an organization, which is determined by the decision and vision of its
management. Most of today's organizations are open systems; therefore, a
continuous fission and fusion is expected in response to the environmental
dynamics.

In nursing home management, on which our discussion centers, there are two broad and interrelated parts that have come to mind: 1) nursing homes as business institutions having many functional parts called departments, and 2) individual resident care management areas designed to ensure a resident's total well-being. To discern the interrelatedness and the goodness-of-fit of the two components, we have utilized a theoretical, historical, and philosophical review of both the traditional and holistic management approaches in the nursing home industry to determine its next logical management approach.

The word *holism* has its roots in the Greek word *holos*, meaning "all," "whole," "entirety," "comprehensive," or "completeness." In medicine, nursing, psychology, philosophy, sociology, metaphysics, and agriculture, the concept of holistic management is widely known, if utilized, but not as much in our business practice. Holistic management is a decision-making and visionary process that comes from the Aristotelian assumption that in all things in nature, the sum of their parts is not necessarily the whole. It is only when individual parts of a system are functional and are connected together to form one entity that they become a whole. Therefore, in making personal or business decisions, it is important that we do not only decide what constitutes the "whole" but also how to ensure that all the parts of the system are functional and dully processed to optimize their performance levels, as we focus on the whole.

However, as we discuss holistic management as a decision-making process, we are reminded of the importance of the concept of the opportunity cost in business and life's choices, and the limitation it can pose on the holistic decision-making. What does an opportunity cost mean and how can it effect a holistic decision-making? In an article titled "What is Opportunity Cost and What Does It Mean for You?" O'Connell (2019) wrote:

> *Opportunity cost is largely defined as a decision you make that alters your personal landscape going forward. Opportunity cost can impact various— and critical—aspects of your life, including money, career, home, family, and other lifestyle elements. In general, it means having to choose one option*

*over the other, be it money, time or lifestyle choices-
and living with the consequences (Wikipedia 2019,
para 1)*

Perhaps you have heard the cliché "there is no free lunch." An
opportunity cost in decision-making means an inescapable fact of life,
which is not necessarily bad but a call for hard work in the world of scarce
resources. In an opportunity cost theory, you will give up something, either
explicitly or implicitly, to achieve something else that is comparatively
better. Since there is no zero opportunity cost in any decision that we
make, it is the principle of holistic management that warns us against
hasty decisions, lack of extra time and precautions to cover enough bases
to enable us to move closer to creating a whole. In other words, in holistic
decision-making, the goal would be to have an opportunity cost that is as
infinitesimal as possible.

We find nursing homes to be such institutions where fragmentation in
care and services can occur and where the holistic management principles
can do some good. Specifically, therefore, the holistic view in nursing home
management emphasizes the belief that the administrator's leadership
of his staff at all levels of the organization becomes the center of that
organizational universe, striving to ensure that all parts of the universe
so created function as one integrated whole toward enhancing regulatory
requirements, quality care for the residents, and the entrepreneurial goals
of the nursing home as a business enterprise.

Nursing home administrators and staffers are in a unique position to
understand, through existing LTC guidelines, the four areas of care that
constitute a resident's universe of needs that must be well coordinated
and delivered to enhance a holistic health and wellness for each resident.
These four areas of care—namely, quality of care, quality of life, resident
environment, and resident funds—will be discussed in the succeeding
pages, needing full understanding by caregivers to be able to deliver care
in the resident-centered care perspective.

In nursing home management, the resident is often considered the
main focal point of that universe. Hence, much of the recent regulatory
discussions toward holistic care in nursing homes have been based on the
concept of "resident-centered care," devoid of any management principles

and approaches inconsistent to producing a holistic outcome for the resident and the organization as a whole. Accordingly, the importance of the other four components associated with the concept of resident-centered care but frequently missing their interconnections must be borne in mind; namely, proper coordination of functional services, proper coordination of resident care plans, proper coordination of resident supervision, and resident engagement.

Proper coordination of functional services as identified in the formulized interdisciplinary team assessment, plan of care, and departmental cooperation is necessary to produce total care and wellness. In nursing homes, it is mandated that each resident receives initial, quarterly, and change-in-condition assessments and plan of care. Embodied in these federal and state laws is that residents' assessments and their plans of care thereof be comprehensive. Residents must receive proper medical, clinical, and nonclinical supervision in an adequate physical and cordial environment for them to survive well. The importance of resident engagement cannot be overstated. It is necessary to ensure that residents, as much as practicable, are afforded full participation and education in the care they receive to empower them to achieve self-motivation, esteem, dignity, independence, and self-care.

For something to be holistic, it must be, in its fullness of being, a scenario that is rooted in many aspects of life, including business management. Holistic management is on the leading edge among the existing management theories, advocating thoroughness and proactivity in decision-making first and foremost. Our decision-making process is key, involving how we manage every aspect of our lives as we interact, either intrapersonally, interpersonally, or extra-personally, within our environments of life.

Like many behavioral theorists, we believe that in all aspects of life there is a positive or negative outcome to our overall human health, wellness, and success based on the state of our psychosocial interactions, which can be normal or abnormal. Holistic management assumes that when our personal or business decisions are fully and duly ordered with clarity in its processes we can achieve our desired outcomes. It also assumes that if the decisions we make do not produce the desired outcome, it must be comprehensively reviewed and corrected. Accordingly, it is fair to infer that if the product we make for human consumption is defective or services we provide are substandard, it all goes back to who made the decision and how much preparation ensued prior to making the decision we implemented. The essence of holistic thinking is even more relevant in the healthcare industry, especially in nursing homes, where zero tolerance for medical error is expected as we must do all we can to avoid pain and suffering for the residents and ourselves.

The concept of holistic management in healthcare first emerged and gained strength under Hippocrates and Florence Nightingale. In business and in politics, it was Allan Savory who brought the philosophy of holism into focus. Hippocrates and Florence Nightingale both believed in "holistic assessment and treatment" of patients. In much the same vein, Kurt Lewin's contribution to the understanding of holistic management stem from his psychological field theory—the gestalt theory and the life span theory, which theorized that a balanced interaction of different parts within a given system or organism was an essential element to its function.

In life span and gestalt theories, it is how well an individual part interacts with the total system and how well adjusted each part is with respect to the whole system. In healthcare management, the implication of these theoretical frameworks on the holistic view of management also has its emphasis on the integration of many health care specialties and systems that exist today to accommodate patients' referrals as may be needed. At a micro level of care, the concept of holism implies that each patient be assessed and treated as a whole person, with the understanding that any defective part is still connected to the whole. For an example, if a patient comes into a clinic complaining of a headache, his doctor and his nurse under holistic medicine are supposed to conduct a holistic assessment of the patient.

It is clear that in nature many animate parts are connected to produce life, which makes seeking a working balance of the human body, soul, and mind an important concept in the holistic approach to medical and nursing practice. The synchronization of these three entities into one is what can psychologically and physiologically produce a well-balanced person. Walter Bradford Cannon (1871–1945) theorized homeostasis and defined it as the necessity for all living things to seek and have internal equilibrium in order to function well. In much the same vein, Freud's theory of the psychic apparatus is a confirmation of the concept of holism in that in order for a human being to function well, the id, the ego, and the superego must work together to ensure balance.

The concept of holistic management in business organizations whose main tenets are decision-making, group participation, inclusiveness, and integration of subparts is no longer limited to the philosophies of Nightingale or Hippocrates for healthcare nursing and medicine, or limited to the Freudian theory of psychic apparatus. The usefulness and application of holistic thinking have expanded to other life's endeavors such as business management, education, land and environmental management.

Critical thinking and effective decision-making are two of the key elements of holistic management. Between 1841 and 1925, Henri Fayol propounded the five functions of management comprising planning, organizing, commanding, coordinating, and controlling. His traditional, hierarchical top-down management model failed to include the importance of critical thinking in decision-making and communication, which are key factors among others to holistic management.

When an organization is designed hierarchically top-down, the locus of decision-making is set to designate who the recipients of that decision would be. Decisions that are only made at the top of the organizational pyramid and intended to be implemented at the lower levels of the pyramid may lose the details of the message on their way down the organizational ladder. Implementing organizational decisions is successful when those slated to implement them hear them from the horse's mouth, or better still, participate in the decision-making process. Holistic management approach does not seek to annul these basic traditional management values but bring them to perfection. And by raising the concerns that have existed with the traditional management approach, today's managers and businessmen are reminded that direct staff participation in decision-making, enhanced by holistic and inclusive management, is about their empowerment and motivation as determinants for overall business success.

For example, Rensis Likert (1903–1981), who propounded systems for management approach in the 1960s favoring group participatory decision-making in an organization, is applauded by proponents of holistic management. Many professional team sport organizations today can be likened to most businesses, where the importance of "who is who" in the organizational hierarchy of authority is oftentimes highlighted while downplaying who does what to create a winning organization. We are imagining a team sport like soccer, American football, and basketball organizations to argue the point relative to who is ultimately important in the organizational structure, and to summarize how holistic management works by recognizing that the input decisions of all organizational members is needed to produce a successful organization—a winning team. Winning in this scenario usually means that when the ball is in the net for a soccer game, basketball, or there has been a touchdown in the case of an American football game, it is often done by the players on the field. In other businesses like nursing homes, it is the first-line staff who are the end users of the holistic management approach to assure the ultimate business success or failure. Like the players on the playing field, it is the first-line staffers in nursing homes who make winning decisions; participating, cooperating, communicating with each other, motivating each other and sharing their skills with each other in order to ensure residents' health and well-being.

In direct healthcare services, a business success or failure is defined as how well a patient has recovered from illness unto creating his well-being, which for the most part depends on the socioclinical and medical contributions of the direct care workers, who are more able to make sound healthcare decision based on their close proximity to the patient. The concept of good decision-making in holistic management supports Stephen Covey's famous quote stating "I am not a product of my circumstances. I am a product of my decisions," which does not necessarily reside in the high echelon of the organization alone.

Peter Drucker (1906–2005), a well-known author and business consultant, devoted a considerable portion of his teaching time to discuss the importance of decision-making, which is considered to be the mainstay in holistic management. According to Drucker, decision-making must be deliberate and linear, comprising classifying the problem, defining the problem, specifying and defining boundary, choosing among alternatives, taking action, and designing feedback. He also advocated three managerial functions that are holistically important and considered to be "managing a business, managing worker and work, and managing the enterprise in community and society." In his book titled *Management*,

Tasks, Responsibilities, Practice, Drucker pointed out two important managerial tasks coinciding with the tenet of holistic management, and wrote:

A manager has two specific tasks. The first is creation of a true whole that

> *is larger than the sum of its parts, a productive entity that turns out more than the sum of the resources put into it . . . a decision or action that satisfies a need in one of these functions by weakening performance in another weakens the whole enterprise. The second specific task of the manager is to harmonize in every decision and action the requirement of immediate and long-range future (Drucker, 1973, 398–399).*

The nursing home industry has faced continued regulatory changes since its inception, most occurring in the last fifty years, with several attempts to improve nursing home quality. But so far it seems regulatory measures alone are unable to produce satisfactory outcomes to squelch the public outcry for a new direction relative to achieving nursing home quality. In the New Testament of the Holy Bible, Jesus warned about putting "new wine into old wineskin" (Luke 5:33–39). He was essentially talking about hanging on to ancient traditions of Judaism, which he considered not only burdensome to his disciples but also outdated, and therefore needed to change. Since that time, the statement has been interpreted more broadly to other areas of human experience. In the contemporary world, it is a call to move from old ways of doing things and embracing new ones.

The foundation of holistic management is a calling to embrace the new thinking and approaches specific to nursing home and business management. Philosophically speaking, the conventional wisdom demands that when we face a small rainfall we use a small umbrella, but when we face a big rainfall, to use a big umbrella to avoid being wet. We believe that it is the new holistic management principles and practices that is key to meeting our present and future personal, health care, and business demands. At a macro-management level, it teaches a comprehensive model of thinking and the decision-making process that ensures the proper method of managing of change within the entrepreneurial and nonentrepreneurial, public or private, for-profit or not-for-profit business enterprises.

In an article titled "The Concept of Holistic Management as a New Approach in the Theory of Management," Porvaznik (2014) noted that "at this point in time, holistic management is only in its infancy. However, its use has already brought indisputable benefit" (Wikipedia 2018, para 7). Holistic management as a decision-making enterprise, involves the importance of recognizing that it takes all functional parts of an organization/business operation, inanimate or animate, to create a holistic operation. This new thinking in management applies to nursing home operations as well. It signals management principles in making business decisions that support interrelationships, efficient interaction of all departments, entities, and persons within the nursing home, including the outside communities it serves. It is noteworthy that in nursing homes, the decisions that we make under holistic management approach oftentimes affect four key operational areas:

- Decisions to connect corporate conglomerates, communities, and stakeholders
- Decisions to connect departmental functions to provide a comprehensive service
- Decisions to ensure that individual residents residing in nursing homes receive comprehensive care based on his/her comprehensive assessment
- Decisions to effectively coordinate issues of resident quality of life, resident quality of care, resident environment, and resident fund management into one holistic care

The responsibility of the holistic decision maker in a nursing home is to ensure that a nursing home achieves its goals and objectives for nursing home quality (NHQ) complying with federal, state, and local regulations and company policies and procedures. According to CMS (Center for Medicare & Medicaid Services), it is the licensed nursing home administrator and the governing body who are assigned the decision-making authority to administer nursing homes, both directly or indirectly reporting to the state government. OBRA '87: F490 to F522 describes the administrative functions of the administrator and the governing body to include their decision-making authority, facility policy development, oversight, education, supervision of material and human resources, and financial management, stating that:

> *The facility must be administered in a manner that enables it to use its resources effectively and efficiently to attain or maintain the highest practicable physical, mental, psychosocial wellbeing of each resident. The facility must have a governing body or a designated person that is legally responsible for establishing and implementing policies regarding the management and operation of the facility* . . . (Terri Pate, Stacy, 2009, "The Facility Guide OBRA Regulations and the long-Term Care Survey Process," P353, MED-PAS, INC.)

One of the frequently asked questions needing an answer relates to reasons why organizations, including nursing homes, should choose the holistic management model as the best business management practice. The partial answer simply lies in the nature of today's concept of globalization, business complexity, competition, regulatory demand, consumers' sophistication and their demand for quality service.

For centuries, many nations have conducted business with one another, traded with each other, bought and sold goods and services nationally and internationally. For thousands of years, trade routes were open for the Chinese, the Indians, and the Japanese. These were regional trade routes. In the same time period, the Greeks also engaged with their Middle Eastern merchants as well, but the biggest multinational business occurred during the periods of the Roman and the British empires, when their political and commercial influence was globally felt. This means that before the start of the twentieth century, organizing and conducting business transactions where goods and services were bought and sold were relatively simple and less complex, with most of them involving simple negotiations or trade by barter. Government regulations and guidelines for business management were almost nonexistent, including the management of almshouses/poorhouses, which later became nursing homes.

But it was the increased number of stories of mistreatments and resident abuse in these institutions that forced government intervention through regulatory means, funding, and oversight. It should be noted that in the past, nursing homes started off as mom and pop operations, sole proprietorships, partnerships, or religious-based owned not-for-profit companies, which were not perceived as lucrative businesses at the time. But with government intervention and funding, a lucrative business enterprise was born, as well as the demand for quality improvement.

Today, many of these nursing home organizations have transformed themselves into mega chain corporations. In the United States, between 2018 and 2020, the top forty-nine nursing home companies had a combined total of 4,034 nursing facilities scattered throughout the country. The industry leader, Genesis Healthcare, alone had 512 facilities, followed by Golden Living with 295 facilities, and HCR Manor Care with 255 facilities.

In order to manage companies whose conglomerates and campuses are located in many different places, with huge distances between them, they must rely on holistic management decisions affecting business planning that leaves no facility or care recipient behind.

The United States is not the only country with nursing homes. All industrialized countries more than ever are now faced with the dilemma of caring for their elderly. They have embraced institutionalized care as well. Today, as we live in a new and complex business and political environment caused by advancements in science and technology, business competition, marketplace expansion, customer demands and expectations, many organizations will be required to make quality decisions that are far reaching to connect with their numerous national and international stakeholders.

Consequently, in an article titled "Holistic Management," managing holistically is viewed as the most effective way to respond to the twenty-first century management functions based on its definition as:

a decision-making framework that assures our decisions are economically, environmentally and socially sound. Holistic management enables you to develop a clear vision of the future you want. Holistic management has its roots in environmental management. But as it is essentially a decision-making process it is applicable to people in all walks of life—households, both rural and urban based businesses, government and educational organizations. By changing the way we make our decisions, we can tackle many of the problems we face (Wikipedia, 2018, para 1).

When Aristotle (384–322 BC) stated that "the whole is greater than the sum of its parts," we have interpreted it to mean that when every individual part in a complex system is included in our decision-making process, the entire system is more worthy. If any part of the system is allowed to be dysfunctional, underutilized, or not utilized at all, the system therefore becomes less worthy of its mission.

Similarly, we see the human body as having many parts and organs to sustain it, but it is only when all of these human parts and organs are functionally engaged that we can declare a person healthy. In most cases, when one human part is dysfunctional or damaged, the entire human system is adversely affected. The example presented on page 18 shows that the five fingers must be a hundred percent functional as a team for the whole hand to function properly.

The concept of holistic management in business owes its origin to a Southern African, Allan Savory, in his quest to solve environmental degradation dating back to 1955. His belief and research cited overpopulation of wild animals such as elephants as the cause for the destruction of the habitat. This restrictive research conclusion led to the government's culling of over 40,000 elephants in that part of Africa in 1969. Savory later regretted the decision that came from his research, calling it the "saddest and greatest blunder of my life" (Wikipedia, 2020, para. 2).

Determined to solve the problem forthrightly, Savory, in his book titled *Holistic Management: A New Decision Making Framework*, developed and advocated for a "holistic framework for decision-making and to holistic planned grazing" (Wikipedia, 2020, para. 2). His professional background includes but is not limited to being a biologist, ecologist, game warden, and an environmentalist. His comparative study on environment in Africa and Texas, USA, also drew an exciting conclusion, dispelling the general belief associated with Africa's poverty. The disparity in the deterioration of the African environment as compared to Texas had nothing to do with land utilization but the quality of the decisions that human managers made affecting these two different environmental situations. Impressed by the outcome of the above study and how promising the holistic management had become, Paddy Reynolds wrote: "Learning to manage holistically, which is of decision-making, I believe should be a life skill practiced by all and taught at schools and understood by law makers. The course has made me optimistic about the future" (Wikipedia, 2018, para 1).

In another article, titled "The Difference a Holistic Business Approach Makes," it is stated:

> *To be a business that uses holistic techniques, it means that the entire organization is considered in its processes and policies as opposed to focusing only on its specific components. By using the holistic approach to running a business, you will make certain that your business is running at its full potential as opposed to simply having strong areas and weak areas . . . this thinking isn't simply "out of the box" but instead it believes that it removes the box altogether (Wikipedia, 2018, para. 1).*

So far, proponents of holistic management, including Allan Savory, believe that the key to the well-being of a business organization lies in the efficacy and quality of the decisions that the decision makers make at every level of the organization. Business decisions that are made with regularity consist of two types of decisions: isolated and recurrent decisions. An isolated decision is a one-time decision relating to business start-ups, business acquisitions, or out of business; while recurrent decisions in business would involve day-to-day operational business issues for which our attention is demanded, such as budgetary controls, renovations, policy change or treatment plans for patients in the case of healthcare services, and employee conflicts. In any of the above situations, the message is the same. Decision-making in holistic management means devoting enough time, resources, research to have a clear and well-defined holistic view of the project.

Benefits of Holistic Management Approach in Organizations

Holistic management provides a useful warning to managers regarding the negative organizational domino effect, whereby a fall of one organizational domino can cause the rest of the dominoes in the chain to fall; consequently calling for due diligence in integrating and nurturing all parts of the organization. A nursing home operation is such an organization in which all parts of the organization and human needs must remain fully functional and comprehensive.

According to an article titled "The Importance of a Holistic Approach to Employee Management," Kuehner-Herbert (2018) viewed the benefits of holistic management from an employee-management perspective, recommending that all employees, especially the frontline staff throughout the entire organization be integrated and provided with staff leadership education, necessary resources, and nurturing that motivate them to perform at higher levels. The assumption is that, for the benefit of a holistic management to abound and help an organization like a nursing home to succeed, the frontline staff must be openly, not imperceptibly, seen as the backbone of resident care. They must be trained to lead the way since other leaders high up in the organizational hierarchy are more likely to be distracted by other organizational issues away from the main goal.

Kuehner-Herbert's emphasis on employee engagement also stems from her belief that:

each worker may perceive a company's goals in their own way depending on their role within the organization, which is why a holistic approach to management is best . . . every part of the organization has a different understanding of the local needs required to serve the global strategy— this explains why organizations that implement holistic management approaches that consider the needs of the whole organization perform better (Wikipedia 2018, para. 1–2).

In general, we have listed below some of the benefits of holistic management that can also be used as measurable goals for the holistic management practitioner to audit his organizational performance. When holistic management is installed, it:

- Encourages a comprehensive assessment of human and organizational conditions for sound decision-making
- Prevents crisis management through group participation
- Assures equitable distribution of company's resources
- Increases staff motivation and morale, involvement, and empowerment
- Creates a strong center-out chain of command in organizational communication
- Creates effective connection among organizational subparts
- Uses trends and innovations evenly across segments of organization
- Creates a systems-thinking process
- Promotes a sustainable organizational growth and regulatory compliance
- Enhances workplace cooperation, collaboration, and teamwork
- Builds a feeling of win/win as a social norm throughout the organization
- Employs the use of first-person plural in organizational failure or success
- Encourages an integrative worldview in management practice; i.e., ability to see the whole picture and think outside the box

- Builds a culture of teamwork
- Helps in managing opportunity cost
- Helps managers to avoid unintended consequences of their actions

In an article titled "A Holistic Approach to Business," Saunders (2007) named the accrued benefits of holistic management in business to include employees' competency, productivity, innovation, and responsiveness, and wrote:

> *Businesses must focus on the holistic approach in order to stay competitive. Most companies have gone lean and mean, which means employees need a broad scope of business knowledge. The era of the narrowly trained specialist seems to be ending. Even the process of developing business managers is changing because businesses require a more versatile approach to innovation and problem-solving (Wikipedia 2020, para 14).*

It is also noteworthy that even though holistic management is not as well known or widely taught as management science in our colleges and universities compared to the principles, concepts, and philosophies of scientific management and humanistic management in managing organizations, it is the holistic management approach that is able to adequately decipher key management principles to respond to change in today's workplace, causing its popularity to increase globally among businesses. Like in climate change debates, even though there is no doubt about the physical evidence of climate change, there is that demand for scientific proof of what is causing it. There are also skeptics who maintain that the earth is taking its normal course and it has nothing to do with human events.

In an article titled "The Business Case for Holistic Management," Lykins (2017) explains some of the skepticisms and the slow recognition of holistic management as well, and pointed out that:

. . . but most of the now 50 years of delay in public and institutional acceptance has been caused by influential academics who state firmly that holistic management is not scientific. Holistic management is 100 percent based on good, sound, long-established scientific principles that no scientist has ever disputed. What holistic management does not have is academic approval from narrowly trained range management experts, who simply cannot see the difference between management that's supported by science and their disapproval of something they do not understand (Wikipedia 2020, para. 15).

A Case for and against Reductionism in Managing Organizations

Organizations that utilize the management systems approach tend to agree that reductionism is the direct opposite of the concept of holism. Having a good understanding of the concept of holism requires a detailed discussion of the concept of reductionism relative to organizations like nursing homes as well. Reductionism is a theoretical concept that favors the breaking down of complex phenomena or systems into its manageable parts for the purpose of identifying and analyzing business success or failure unit by unit without exploring the effect of the connection existing between one unit of operation and the other, or the mega system. As defined in a management literature titled "Reductionism x Management," "holism and reductionism are two opposing approaches in the theory of systems that are used also in the theory of management. Holism explores the whole, the entire system . . . reductionism reduces the system's exploration toward understanding its key parts" (Wikipedia 2018, para.1).

As much as we idealize the holistic management approach in organizations, nothing precludes reductionism from having an effective interaction with holism to meet specific organizational objectives, and nothing therefore precludes organizations from utilizing both concepts at different times as projects necessitate, as long as in the end holism is the dominant concept to guide the entire organization. Reductionism will not negate the holistic values in organizations if it serves as an alternative means to independently evaluate each part of the organization as it recognizes the connection of each part of the organization to other parts to make one whole.

In nursing homes, which are usually managed through departmentalization as designated in its organizational chart, holism and reductionism can coexist. However, the tradition that some departments in nursing homes are more critical or more valuable than others in resident care and caring is debatable under holistic management. The false assumption made by some care providers is that certain care contributions from some health care disciplines are more worthy than others, and that one is subsidiary to the other, is not supported by the holistic principles. Such a reductionist thinking may be the cause of noncompliance or inconsistent compliance to the F-tags and K-tags. Federal and state inspections are designed to review each nursing home as a whole, and residents must receive a comprehensive care.

Over the years, for example, the nursing department in nursing homes has been viewed as the most consequential department among approximately nine other departments that constitute a nursing home. Such conclusion was based on the reductionist shortsightedness and "oversimplification" of organizational systems, with the tendency of not being evenhanded with all parts of the system. Strict reductionism has been criticized for the possibility of creating a discriminatory practice among departments when competing for scarce resources, as well as interdepartmental favoritism, especially if senior leaderships or supervisors have prior educational or business affiliations with them.

Reductionism is also noted for placing artificial boundaries and limitations within organizations, and therefore limiting humans from imagining their future growth and development. There was a time when quality of care for nursing and medical services was considered key to resident care satisfaction in nursing homes. The reality is, besides the quality of care domain, there are three other quality domains, consisting of quality of life, resident environment, and resident fund management. OBRA '87 recognizes that all service domains are equally important to achieve the resident's total well-being. In this case, this principle of subsidiarity involving departmental functions and services has so far produced a defeatist and false sense of superiority or inferiority, producing lack of effective cooperation among parts in holistic management. In an article titled "Defining Quality of Care," Harris-Wehling (1990.1) wrote, "Not all goals of the patient's care are technical or scientific in nature.

Non-medical goals such as patient satisfaction and consistency with patient preferences are considered to be of importance and a critical dimension of quality care for the elderly."

It is noteworthy therefore how much the concepts of "resident centered care" and "comprehensive care" have transformed the meaning of quality care and provided new dimensions as to how convoluted it can be to try to interpret the beginning, the end, or the complementary relationship between holism and reductionism in the management of nursing homes. While we insist that care providers follow their comprehensive care protocols in the assessment and treatment of residents, they must also apply resident-centered care protocols to assess and treat residents in accordance with their individuality and needs preferences, assuring that each department in a nursing home has a designated service it must provide.

It should be noted that the nursing home is one of those organizations where a failure in one department is likely to affect one or two departments, and indeed the whole system. The effect of the intersection between reductionism and holism in managing both the direct resident care and day-to-day operation of the entire nursing home must be reviewed. Therefore, there is a need for care providers in nursing homes to be eclectic, dynamic, and flexible in their management style in order to succeed well in a service-oriented industry where there tends to be no "one-size fit all" in services.

Holistic business management is about the holistic management of human behavior, their technical skills, their motivation, attitudes, and perceptions as they affect the organizational goals as a whole, as rooted in holistic management principles. In an article titled "The Importance of Behavioral Science in Business Management," Siddiqui (2015) stated "the behavioral science is of great importance to a business management . . . it deals with human culture and human development" (Wikipedia, 2020, para 1).

After the Industrial Revolution (1760–1840), many management theories were developed to help the emergent manufacturing industry increase productivity, economic efficiency, workers' well-being, and the prosperity of all mankind. In the 1900s, it was Frederick Taylor who introduced the theory of scientific management into the world of business management. In the tradition of reductionism, this theory emphasized the concepts of rationalization, specialization, departmentalization, and standardization. Production efficiency was also achieved through system fragmentation, meaning the breaking of the organization into manageable chunks, and rigidity of standards in the era of man versus machine.

In much the same vein, Max Weber (1864–1920) advocated bureaucratic systems administered and conducted only by trained professionals, who would either formulate or follow strict rules and standards. Scientific management, whose offspring is reductionist management, has its advantages and disadvantages, but it is its disadvantages that has opened new doors to other management theories such as the holistic management approach, emphasizing integrative, unitary, and humanistic approach to management.

Consequently, Frederick Herzberg (1923–2000) became famous in theorizing the two-factor theory of hygiene and motivational factors, focusing on what the causes of staff satisfaction or dissatisfaction were. Elton Mayo (1880–1949), with his landmark studies at Hawthorne, was another theorist who advocated the human relation movement. He theorized that in any workforce, there is a coexistence of an informal alongside a formal organization that has to be holistically managed.

In the era of humanistic psychology was also Abraham Maslow (1908–1970), who theorized that human beings have needs, which are hierarchically arranged from lower level needs to upper level needs, that must be satisfied hierarchically upward. Douglas McGregor is the author of *The Human Side Enterprise* and the theorist of Theory X and Theory Y, devoted to analyzing human motivation. The chronology in the humanistic management theories has assured that human beings are in an era where organizational members are expected to view all aspects of organizations through one microscope to see it as one whole. Conversely, there is that realization that when managers do not see or act on the "big picture," some parts of the organization can be neglected or overlooked, resulting in its singular demise or the demise of the organization as a whole.

Now, how can piecemeal work become a useful part of holistic management, especially in nursing homes? When piecemeal work was first introduced in the 1500s under the guild system unto the Industrial Revolution period and adopted as part of the scientific management theory of Frederick Winslow Taylor, its advantages were only linked to the concepts of the division of labor, job specialty, easy measurement of employee productivity levels, pay rates, and economic benefits to the employer. Additionally, pay rates of employees were easily matched with their final pay for producing more or less pieces of work. The psycho-philosophical and economic impact of piecemeal work, which means bit by bit or one piece at a time, was not envisioned, and has not been totally reviewed to this day. As a result, piecemeal work has prevailed in most of our industries, including nursing homes, for over 500 years.

Some of the criticisms of piecemeal work can be seen as producing lack of cohesion and connectivity among organizational subparts and unity of purpose, preventing each employee in his own cocoon to perceive the big organizational picture, let alone conceive how a completed project was all brought together, of which he was, nevertheless, a part. The after effect of disintegration or piecemeal work is low employee motivation resulting from their inability to claim an adequate feeling of ownership at each project's completion.

With regards to nursing homes, and despite the recommendation of a comprehensive assessment and treatment of residents, most work performed in nursing homes are in fact piecemeal due to employees' specialization by training and division of labor. For example, each classification of nursing staff—namely, GNAs, LPNs, and RNs—is allowed to only receive resident-related work assignments in accordance with his/her skill set, hoping that in the end, when all contributions are put together, it will all amount to whole. It is noteworthy that as the holistic nursing management seeks to move nursing home workers to see all care areas as being interconnected to produce total resident well-being, there is a correlation existing between piecemeal work assignments and piecemeal thinking constituting an impediment to achieving comprehensive care for the residents. As discussed earlier, the goal of holistic management is to connect all parts to one functional whole. But if staff are locked into their own specialized areas of work and thoughts, the utopia of achieving the whole is unlikely to exist.

Fundamentals of Holistic Resident-Centered Care in Holistic Nursing Home Management

The holistic model of resident care in nursing is a comprehensive model believed to be at the center of the discipline of nursing care (Zamanzadeh, Jasemi, Valizadeh, Keogh, and Taleghani, 2015). Holistic care involves the recognition of a person as a whole, and supports the interrelationships of an individual's social, biological, psychological, and spiritual needs. It includes a wide range of strategies that include education, medication, self-help, communication, and complementary and alternative medicine or CAM (Zamanzadeh et al., 2015).

Holistic care strives to maintain human dignity. The relationship between caregivers and patients is based on respect, equality, and reciprocity, where patients participate in the decision-making processes of their care. The goal of holistic care is to enhance the depth of understanding of caregivers with regards to patient's total needs through a comprehensive care plan on admission.

The discharge requirement of residents with comorbidity further dramatizes the importance of the holistic approach to care, requiring that such residents are not ready for discharge until a comprehensive wellness is declared by a health professional or the resident personal doctor. In recent years, through government oversight, the acute care hospitals and nursing homes have been cooperating in the effort to ensure that rehospitalization of nursing home residents due to a premature discharge is practicably avoidable.

Before the concept of holistic care in healthcare by Florence Nightingale and Hippocrates Asclepiades, what was prevalent was a piecemeal management treatment of diseases limited to nursing and medical practice. Nurses are often known to be the front-end care givers, but their adaptation of holistic care has continued to be a slow process, leading to the neglect of important aspects of patients' health conditions. In an article titled "Effective Factors in Providing Holistic Care: A Quantitative Study," V. Zamanzadeh et al. (2015) confirmed that "unfortunately, there is compelling evidence that most nurses have been educated with a biomedical allopathic focus and do not have a good understanding of the meaning of holistic care" (Wikipedia 2020, para. 5).

CAM, palliative care, recognition of spiritual needs, and treatment of psychological factors such as depression and anxiety are all examples of holistic care that improves the quality of life of nursing home residents. Unfortunately, most nurses are educated in the medical-centered model of care rather than the patient-centered holistic model. According to Zamanzadeh et al. (2015), studies that addressed holistic care in the US found that only 33 percent of patients receive holistic care, and a study performed in England showed that only 5 percent of patients received holistic care. Nursing homes in the United States must also be evaluated based on our illustration on pg 127 of this book.

There are numerous benefits to the utilization of holistic care, including self-confidence and self-awareness in patients; a better understanding of the correlation of the mind, body, and spirit among caregivers; and includes every nursing practice that involves the treatment of the whole person. It is noteworthy for health practitioners to pay attention to the buzzword from the recipients of care. They expect total wellness, which is implicit in holistic care, and as is documented in the article "Medical Conditions of Nursing Home Admissions." It is stated that "the reason for admission to long-term nursing home (NH) care is often a combination of factors . . . reflected by health status, disease and functional disability and basic Activities of Daily Living (ADL)" (Wikipedia 2018, para 2).

Holistic nursing, particularly for patients admitted into nursing homes, goes beyond the typical concentration on BMES: bingo, medication, eat, and sleep. And beyond the six recommended areas by CMS for declines in ADLs; namely, eating, bathing, getting dressed, toileting, transferring, and continence. A holistic nurse or physician must be engaging with his individual patient in ways that enable him to see his patient as a whole person worthy of laughing with, empathizing with, spending quality time with, and receiving care beyond the patient's physical-medical needs. The holistic nurse must concern himself with what defines his patient as a whole person to include his emotions, spirituality, preferences, culture, and socialization, to name a few.

Adopting a patient-centered holistic framework of care in nursing homes has great beneficial effects on both the patient and the nurse or caregiver. Caregivers are motivated when they see their patients thrive, and are therefore entitled to more resources, more time, and less caseloads to be successful under their new mandate. Caregivers are generally trained to do no harm. By design, caregivers work diligently to do good at all times to get positive outcomes; and with the application of holistic approach to care, nothing can be more redemptive.

In recent years, medical research, medical breakthroughs, and medical statistical findings are validating holistic care as the best option for care givers. The definition of healthcare quality itself is an excellent example. IOM (Institute of Medicine) has defined quality care as "the degree to which health services for individuals and populations increase the likelihood of desired health outcomes and consistent with current professional knowledge" (Wikipedia, 2018 para.1). It is within this 1986 definition that care standards and measurements were developed and expanded for acute and long-term care services. Accordingly, quality healthcare would be assessed and measured based on safety, effectiveness, patient-centeredness, timeliness, efficiency, and equitability.

The comparison between traditional versus holistic approaches to medical and nursing services, delineating benefits for patients, clarifies why there is a need to embrace a holistic approach to care and caring for patients in all care centers. According to an article titled "Traditional Nursing Vs Holistic Nursing," Darson (2013) defined the difference between traditional and holistic care, and concluded that "Holistic nursing is broadly defined as using nursing knowledge and practices in conjunction with other psychological, spiritual, social, interpersonal, and biological skills to treat the whole patient as in mind, body, and spirit (in contrast to traditional nursing, which only focuses on treating the medical condition)"(Wikipedia 2018 para 1).

Other factors supporting holistic care are varied. In 1970, the method and process of looking at, diagnosing, and treating human diseases when they are multiple was revolutionized. The concept of comorbidity was introduced by a doctor, epidemiologist, and researcher, Alvan R. Feinstein. Dr. Feinstein's message was clear that human diseases cannot be treated in isolation, and that in medicine, besides the primary disease, secondary diseases must receive a concurrent assessment and treatment as well. Comorbidity in medicine therefore is defined as "the presence of one or more additional or disorders co-occurring with . . . a primary disease or disorder; in the countable sense of the term, a comorbidity . . . is each additional disorder or disease. The additional disorder may, also, be a behavioral or mental disorder" (Wikipedia, 2018 para.1).

The degree to which the reality and prevalence of comorbidity/ multimorbidity conditions have impacted the overall patients' health today is echoed in the World Health Organization (WHO) project declarations on the prevention and treatment of chronic diseases. Notable is its disappointing 2002 World Health Report as contained in the report titled "Integrated Chronic Disease Prevention and Control," predicting worsened global "mortality, morbidity, and disability" due to an increase in chronic diseases currently accounting to 60 percent. They predicted that "by 2020 their contribution is expected to rise to 73% of all deaths . . ." (Wikipedia 2018, para 1).

Today, many patients admitted into acute or long-term care settings are known to have comorbid or multimorbid conditions that health-care professionals cannot ignore. The effective way of tackling comorbid or multimorbid pathologies begins with the care providers' holistic mindset alongside clinical competence in dealing with different subject matters of medicine and nursing. "Comorbidity is widespread among the patients admitted at multidiscipline hospitals" (Comorbidity, Wikipedia, 2018, para 1) and in nursing homes.

In a research study titled "Patterns of Chronic Co-morbid Medical Conditions in Older Residents of US Nursing Homes: Differences between the Sexes and Across Age span," Moore et al. (2015) stated that "hypertension, vascular disease, dementia, arthritis, depression and gastro-esophageal reflux disease were part of the most prevalent co-morbid conditions. Multi-morbidity patterns can be identified in nursing home residents and vary with age and by sex" (Wikipedia, 2018 para 2).

The Van den Brink et al. (2012) research on "Resident with Mental-Physical multi-morbidity living in long-term care facilities: Prevalence and Characteristics. A Systematic Review" concluded that "although exact figures are lacking, mental-physical multi-morbidity is common in LTC residents . . . multi-morbidity is defined as the simultaneous occurrence of several medical conditions in the same person" (Wikipedia 2018 para 1). The prevalence of multimorbid cases currently found in nursing homes require a multidimensional response involving diverse healthcare disciplines and specialties nevertheless working cohesively as a team for their common goal—the patient's health and wellbeing.

In 2016, Centers for Medicaid & Medicare services (CMS) handed down updated rulings and methods on resident care plans from its 1991 mandates, consistent with the spirit of holistic medical and nursing care. In an article titled "Federal Requirements of Participation for Nursing Homes Issued September 2016 Summary of Key Changes in the Rule Part 2," the emphasis noted is on the definitions of "comprehensive care plans," "the interdisciplinary team," and "comprehensive person-centered care planning" (Wikipedia 2018 para 2). It is noteworthy that in these rulings, CMS emphasizes an interdisciplinary as opposed to multidisciplinary team approach, since the latter has been discredited for lacking integration as a key ingredient among team members and their disciplines to achieve an effective and holistic health outcome that adequately reflects an individual patient's total care needs.

Accordingly, each nursing home must develop policies and procedures to assist them in achieving this goal. It must be noted that the resident's comprehensive assessment is an important first step toward developing a holistic treatment plan. In much the same vein, each nursing home must assure the efficacy and integrity of each comprehensive assessment, comprehensive person-centered care plan by retaining professionals qualified to get the job done.

Outside organizations who do not only agree, embrace, and support holistic approach in medical and nursing services but also act as resource factories and support systems for in-service education, general education, change in school curricula, and public knowledge on the subject matter are many. Typical among the oldest of these organizations are the American Holistic Medical Association (AHMA) and the American Nurses Association (ANA), with the goal of propagating a holistic approach to medical and nursing services as opposed to the traditional approach. They "advocate for the use of holistic and integrative medicine by all licensed healthcare providers" (Wikipedia 2018, para 1).

In an article titled "Skilled Nursing Facilities and Other Long Term Care Facilities: Addressing Issues of Cost and Quality," Nochomovitz (n d.) assessed the services provided in nursing homes as varied and multidimensional, implying a holistic management of resident care, and wrote "long-term care as it exists today is broad in its definition and generally refers to a range of services that supports the daily needs of individuals with limited functioning or disability" (Wikipedia 2018, para 1). Accordingly, while there may be differences among healthcare facilities (acute, long-term care, and assisted living) based on levels of care, their main similarity is a focus on "safety, quality of care, and best patients' outcomes" (Nochomovitz).

Chapter 3

Management Theories: Toward
Achievement of Nursing Home Quality

From time immemorial, dating back to Hippocrates and Nightingale, optimizing healthcare quality has remained the highest priority for healthcare providers. Having a worldview of the industry you are in, personal philosophy, knowledge of company policy, knowledge of scientific theories and management concepts, is what produces management effectiveness that optimizes quality.

Research shows that most nursing homes and other healthcare organizations have been presented or have experimented with some of the available clinical and management theories, quality assurance tools and concepts designed not only to improve but also to sustain healthcare quality in nursing homes. Managing a large-scale and complex nursing home organization to assure quality care for all patients is a serious undertaking. However, it is our observation that incumbents, mostly nurses in management positions, in nursing homes are not only performing dual functions but are expected to have a knowledge base that is both clinical and managerial. Whether fusing two distinct skill sets in one incumbent is a good idea or not is debatable. But by blurring the professional line separating the clinical from managerial functions, there may be some who may see the idea as creating "Jacks of all trades, master of none."

It is noteworthy that nursing homes are noted for being labor intensive and clinical intensive, for which providing an effective employee supervision to ensure quality care can be overwhelming. Therefore, the familiarity with clinical and management theories applicable to different work-related circumstances has become critical in nursing homes, demanding a professional acumen, which tends to be in short supply, or cause the fulfilling of the Peter Principle in terms of new innovations to improve nursing home quality.

Since OBRA '87, the nursing home industry has come under an increased pressure for change. The affected areas are in the staffing ratios for nurses, proof of continuing education, proof of quality standard measurement and government surveillance, to name a few. The choice and qualification for internal staff supervisory management is always the company's decision, sometimes leading to management by one-size-fits-all in a complex organizational system where employee supervision can be key to quality. Because nursing homes generally have variability in work style and assignments between diverse staff, and residents with different health needs, behavior characteristics, cultures, preferences, and family demands, establishing a single optimizing organizational goal has been problematic. Not having a well-defined supervisory management plan for the diverse areas of care has affected compliance.

The expected solution is for nursing assistants, for example, to have supervisors who are hands-on and designated only to supervise them. In nursing homes, managers themselves must learn to be more eclectic in the use of their management skills, prevailing concepts, theories, and approaches to holistic management in their day-to-day operation. In an organization like the nursing home, it is the quality of staff supervision that is likely to result in a well-organized and productive workforce where compliance is possible.

In a book titled *Social Style/Management Style: Developing Productive Work Relationships*, Bolton and Bolton (1984, vii) suggested that "the ability to understand and relate to different working styles is one of the most useful ways of forging effective work relationships." The use of a social-style concept seems promising in workplaces like the nursing home in that it is "nonthreatening . . . easy to learn and relatively easy to apply."

Achieving nursing home quality has continued to be an important concern in our societies in the last few years. Selecting appropriate strategies and approaches to achieving the desired nursing home quality is critical, usually requiring a committed leadership and a stick-to-it attitude in all levels of management and staff throughout the organization, including corporate support.

Some of the immediate and relevant management concepts designed to help improve nursing home quality are provided:

Total Quality Management

Integrating holistic methods into traditional management approaches, including total quality management (TQM), allows for a more complete model of nursing home administration (Johannsen, 2013). Holistic medical care is a philosophy that stresses that the whole is greater than the sum of all its parts, and that healthcare services should focus on every aspect of an individual, including their psychological, social, and physical needs (Zamanzadeh, Jasemi, Valizadeh, Keogh, and Taleghani, 2015). TQM is considered a holistic management approach that is utilized to maintain the sustainability of improvements that are made in the total performance of the nursing home (Alimohammadlou and Eslamloo, 2016).

Total quality management (TQM) is defined as "a management philosophy concerned with people and work processes that focus on customer satisfaction and improves organizational performance" (Al-Shdaifat, 2015). After its creation in the 1980s in Japan, TQM was prominent in the business sector among organizations wishing to improve the development of their companies. While the theory of TQM has been suggested in principle to be effective, its application by businesses has not resulted in improvements in their performance (Mosadeghrad, 2012). Studies have shown that there is a failure rate as high as 95 percent in businesses that have used this approach to improve performance rates.

Implementing TQM in healthcare is even more difficult than in business due to its special characteristics (Mosadeghrad, 2012). The fundamental principles that influence TQM include identifying and compiling problems, managing processes, averting mistakes, and creating targeted goals (Vituri and Evora, 2015). As a management model in healthcare, TQM has been controversial among researchers regarding its effectiveness. Mosadeghrad (2012) states that TQM requires a large time commitment that does not always produce beneficial results, and he has proposed a quality management model for healthcare organizations that will help managers effectively make changes to improve internal processes.

In order to effectively integrate TQM into an organization, there needs to be a clear understanding of its principles (Mosadeghrad, 2012). There are a number of obstacles in healthcare that have to be overcome in order to implement TQM, which include lack of top management support, the departmentalized and organizational hierarchy found in healthcare, insufficient employee training and involvement, and professional autonomy. Mosadeghrad (2012) suggests a new model for healthcare organizations called strategic collaborative quality management (SCQM) that combines the principles of TQM, strategic management, and project management. The ultimate goal of SCQM is to improve the quality of services offered by the nursing home, as well as a better, practical understanding for managers of quality management (Mosadeghrad).

Appreciative Inquiry

Appreciative inquiry (AI) takes a different approach to change than most frameworks because it employs positive inquiry and questions to explore the values that both individuals and team members share in order to implement the best practices of the organization (Moorer et al., 2017). The insights that are gained from the inquiries are used to develop a vision that builds on the strengths of the organization in order to create a management plan. That vision is then developed through designing management processes and systems that corroborate the organization's strengths, ethics, and performance patterns. An advantage to utilizing AI as a framework for change is that it focuses on the positive aspects (what is working) of the issue being researched rather than the problems and how to fix them. When focusing on the negative or problems, employees become discouraged and disempowered (Moorer et al.).

When initiating an AI in a nursing home, both the top management administrators and the front-line employees (nurses, aides, nurse managers, security, and environmental services) have to be involved at the same time (Moorer et al., 2017). Once a topic is chosen (more effective management in nursing homes), the stages when performing an AI can be initiated: discover, dream, design, and destiny (Kessler, 2013). The dream stage focuses on interviewing each participant and what they consider to be their own "best of" story regarding the chosen topic. Everyone should be equally engaged. These stories are collected and explored before moving to the dream stage. In the dream stage, participants are asked to imagine their organization as the best in relation to the topic. The design phase involves participants developing specific proposals for the change in the organization. Finally, in the destiny stage, the role of the manager or administrator is to monitor the novel changes that they want to enhance, and then create processes that will encourage change (Kessler).

Lean Supply Chain Management

Lean supply chain management (LSCM) evolved from the Toyota Motor Company's model of production systems during the last decade (Teich and Faddoul, 2013). The issues of manufacturing and technology problems were found to be universal factors that affected management and could be transferred to healthcare management systems. LSCM is a diverse, multifaceted concept that necessitates the application of multiple dimensions at the same time. Because of the commitment required and the impact on all levels of the organization, managers will have to make an assessment regarding whether the company is ready to proceed with such an enormous change (Teich and Faddoul).

Before looking at the successes created by LSCM, obstacles and failures need to be examined, which will give the organization an idea of how to develop their strategies for change (Teich and Faddoul, 2013). Some of the barriers to success include the absence of senior management commitment, no autonomy of the team, poor communication, and no conviction by employees of LSCM. Teich and Faddoul (2013) found that there was a common theme in lessons learned and "that organizations need to change at a behavioral and cultural level and this should be translated directly into an endless process of continuous improvement."

The application of LSCM in healthcare can also be implemented in a holistic manner by transforming an overall management strategy (Lawal et al., 2014). There has not been a plethora of research on the application of LSCM and its sustainability in healthcare. The majority of studies have found that implementation of LSCM has been successful, but there has not been much documentation concerning obstacles when utilized in healthcare. Therefore, information concerning its use in health care, especially the effects it may have on holistic management practices and outcomes in nursing homes (Lawal et al.).

Six Sigma

Six Sigma and LSCM are two of the most popular management frameworks utilized in continuous improvement programs (Mousa, 2013). Six Sigma was developed by the Motorola Corporation and uses an approach known as DMAIC (define, measure, analyze, improve, and control), as well as statistical tools to determine root causes of an issue and to decrease any variations. When combining the two frameworks, there is a philosophy that encompasses powerful statistical tools that solve the issues at hand and create rapid improvements with reduced costs (Mousa).

Six Sigma is a "statistical measure of defect rate within a system supported by statistical techniques" (Mousa, 2013). The use of Six Sigma in healthcare was initiated in the 1990s because defects, mistakes, and incidents are widespread in healthcare (Buttigieg, Dey, and Gauci, 2015). The question "Are human systems so different from others in which Six Sigma has been achieved or attempted that high levels of reliability are unattainable?" posed by Mark Chassin encouraged the adoption of the framework (Buttigieg et al).

The use of Six Sigma principles is a strategy that healthcare organizations can adopt to achieve operational and financial performance improvement. Today, reducing waste and decreasing costs in healthcare organizations have become a major priority precipitating the focus of lean management and Six Sigma on determining ways to decrease spiraling health-care costs, improving quality, and decreasing waste (Buttigieg et al., 2015).

Quality Assurance and Performance Improvement

The quality assurance and performance improvement (QAPI) program is one of the latest management concepts being experimented with in nursing homes across America to enhance nursing home quality (NHQ). In OBRA '87, the designation for quality assurance, a.k.a. quality assurance and performance improvement is 483.75(o) F520. It is hoped that through QAPI all resident care services and staff services will be comprehensively examined quarterly at the minimum. In this sense, we see QAPI as the one area of nursing home practice in close proximity to holistic management.

QAPI in nursing homes was strengthened by the landmark health reform legislation signed into law by President Barack Obama in 2010 known as the Affordable Care Act (ACA), Patient Protection Affordable Care Act (PPACA) or Obamacare. In 2011, the Center for Medicare and Medicaid Services (CMS) imposed QAPI on nursing homes not only as another mandated nursing home program but as a requirement for participation in the Medicare and Medicaid program starting in 2016. In an article titled "QAPI Description and Background," it is stated that:

> *The Secretary (delegated to CMS) shall establish and implement a QAPI program for facilities that include development of standards (regulations) and provision of technical assistance on the development of best practices in order to meet such standards. This new provision significantly expands the level and scope of required QAPI activities to ensure that facilities continuously identify and correct quality deficiencies as well as sustain performance improvement (Wikipedia p1, 2018).*

It is noteworthy that QAPI is driven by three principles: data collection activities, data analysis, and corrective action. The questions often raised by opponents of QAPI are threefold: 1) Is the QAPI program reactive rather than proactive, diminutive rather than comprehensive as its framers intended? 2) Is the QAPI program holistic enough in its approach to improve nursing home quality, and 3) how easy and practical is the QAPI program to be implemented and sustained? Answers to these questions are not likely to be known until the full schedule of QAPI implementation is completed in November 2019. Needless to say, there may be an additional time period needed thereafter to assess the felt strength and weaknesses of QAPI.

Nevertheless, since the inception of QAPI in nursing homes, its scope has expanded by state and federal agencies stipulating that QAPI be implemented in three phases, with phase 1 starting in November 2016, phase2 in November 2017, and phase 3 in November 2019. Additionally, in an article titled "What Are QAPI Programs in Long-Term Care," Kluwer (2017) clarified the stipulation that each facility "must develop a QAPI plan by November 2017 and submit to the Survey Agency at their annual recertification survey" (Wikipedia 2019, para. 2).

Nursing facilities do not have the option to opt out of QAPI, hence their regulatory compliance can be estimated at 100 percent even though its use and outcome effect may be questionable. They oftentimes lack operational consistency. Most nursing facilities have QAPI policy manuals that are usually buried among other books in the administrator's office, only to be found when the facility realizes that the QAPI meeting has been missed for several months, QAPI minutes are not current, or some survey is approaching.

However, proponents of QAPI have maintained that as a management tool, QAPI is poised for success, advocating that QAPI be treated with the seriousness it deserves. They argue that because the program has two complementary components—the QA and the PI merged together—its capability to help prevent deficient practices or waste in nursing homes is strengthened.

The QA portion of the QAPI program establishes standards of expected quality or outcome measures, while the PI portion of the QAPI program mandates and encourages a continuous study of processes for the purpose of improving future outcomes and services for nursing homes. They also have cited the efficacy of QAPI to include increase in staff technical and clinical skills to help them solve quality problems, creating opportunities for staff to pursue new goals and enhancing increased staff motivation and self-fulfillment to provide better care for residents.

The goal of QAPI in nursing homes is to "establish, implement effective, comprehensive, data-driven QAPI programs that focus on systems of care including indicators of outcomes of care, quality of life, and resident and staff satisfaction" (Kluwer 2017,1). Rubertino (2014), referring to QAPI, states "improving quality of care reaches beyond the basics of gathering statistics in a quality assessment and assurance (QAA) meeting and monitoring only our quality measures retrospectively."

There are five key elements and twelve action steps in a QAPI program that its leaders and participants must master for effective implementation and management of QAPI. The five key elements of QAPI are listed as follows: 1) design and scope; 2) governance and leadership; 3) feedback, data systems, and monitoring; 4) performance improvement project; and 5) Systematic analysis and action.

In an article titled "QAPI Basics—The Five Elements and 12 Steps," Leatherbarrow (2016, 3) listed the twelve action steps of QAPI as:

> *1) leadership responsibility and accountability, 2) develop a deliberate approach to teamwork, 3) take your "pulse" with self-assessment, 4) identify your organization's guiding principles, 5) develop your QAPI plan, 6) conduct a QAPI awareness campaign, 7) develop a strategy for collecting and using data, 8) identify your gap and opportunities, 9) prioritize quality opportunities and charter PIP, 10) plan, conduct and document PIPs, 11) getting to the "root" of the problem, 12) take systemic action*

In spite of the perceived and commonly cited benefits of QAPI in nursing home operations, most nursing homes do face difficulties in establishing, implementing, or managing QAPI programs consistently with the full five key elements and the twelve action steps in place. A successful QAPI program that includes all key elements and action steps requires hard work, dedication, sufficient and trained staff, consistent leadership, time commitment, and full participation. QAPI meetings need to be conducted on a routine schedule with participants who are enthusiastic and well prepared, with reports and assigned responsibilities.

These are some of the internal organizational qualities and resources that are in high demand to make QAPI successful, but unfortunately, in short supply in most nursing homes. QAPI programs in nursing homes also tend to lack an active, consistent bottom-up staff participation in practice. Strong corporate support is needed beyond providing lip-service and a written policy.

In an article titled "QAPI: Nursing Challenges and Successes," Flanagan (2017, 1) pointed out why the proactive, preventive, longitudinal care planning effect, as well as the comprehensive nature, as promised in QAPI may be eroding in nursing homes, and wrote:

> *The first two elements of the QAPI process-design and scope, and governance and leadership remain a challenge for many centers. The average tenure for director of nursing is 2.5 to 3 years with an average turnover rate of 47%. Nursing home administrators have a similar trajectory. The turnover rate makes it difficult for centers to keep QAPI teams motivated and cohesive. Each new leader may have a different focus or vision, and some leaders can be shortsighted and only focus on deficiencies rather than on a long-term vision for success.*

Based on the existing internal organizational concerns, the nursing home industry can benefit from evaluating not only how proactive, comprehensive, holistic, longitudinal, and practical its QAPI is, but also how much QAPI has thus far served the community to help improve the NHQ. QAPI, which was introduced in 2011, is relatively a new initiative within the nursing home industry. To ensure the benefit of QAPI as a reliable nursing home quality achievement tool (NHQAT) of the future, nursing homes would need to invest a considerable amount of time in staff education, staff motivation and their continuous education, adequately designed to enhance proper learning to practicalize QAPI.

In 1956, Benjamin Bloom theorized a learning process that must be hierarchical upward from knowing, comprehending, applying, analyzing, synthesizing, and evaluating. This step-by-step learning process from the lower learning difficulty to the higher ones is to assure that learners achieve their learning goals enthusiastically and with good retention. Bloom Taxonomy is noted for classifying "educational learning objectives into levels of complexities and specificity" (Wikipedia 2018, para.1).

Regarding which educational model can help in advancing QAPI, John Dewey also advocated the concept of the "progressive education," stating "progressive education is essentially a view of education that emphasizes the need to learn by doing." Dewey believed that human beings learn through a "hands-on approach" (Wikipedia 2018, para 1).

Already noted for crisis management due to competing healthcare delivery demands; struggling with issues of regulatory compliance, staff shortages; inadequate staff training, budget; and meeting the bottom line, to name a few, nursing homes, unlike the auto industry, never found the time or the effort to establish its own quality assurance/control model that is not externally imposed.

The hierarchical top-down initiative, from the federal government ACA to CMS, unto nursing homes requiring a considerable amount of human resources and energy for staff education, staff motivation, staff participation, data collection, recordkeeping, and consistent QAPI leadership can be seen as cause for accepting QAPI grudgingly in nursing homes. In much the same vein, there tends to be an incongruent expectation between the framers and the end users of QAPI, questioning the worthiness of QAPI, which in the end could mean that as a nursing home quality achievement tool (NHQAT), QAPI, by design, may not be holistic enough to produce nursing home quality. It can also mean that its failure to assure nursing home compliance lies somewhere else.

Structure-Process-Outcome (SPO)

Avedis Donabedian (1919–2000) is known as the father of quality assurance in health care. He developed his quality care framework in 1966, calling it the Donabedian Model. The model quality achievement is represented linearly by three separate box containers of structure, process, and outcomes—in that order. In the structure box, the manager determines what materials of production are needed to render an effective service (staff, financial and equipment, supplies skill set, and so forth). The process box denotes how those materials are effectively used to optimize outcome, and outcome represents the effect of the service on the client.

The one criticism that exists is that the model is too linear, but proponents applaud it because the framework is easy to use, can be used to modify structures and processes within the healthcare system if necessary. For these reasons, the Donabedian structure-process-outcome model has been known to be more effective than other quality of care frameworks in assessing the quality of healthcare.

In an article titled "Donabedian's Lasting Framework for Health Care Quality," Ayanian and Markel (2016) acknowledged Donabedian's proposal of using "the triad of structure, process and outcome to evaluate the quality of healthcare. That triad, along with his seven pillars of quality continues to inform efforts to improve care."

In an article titled "The Seven Pillars of Quality," Donabedian (1990) outlined what he considered the seven pillars of quality in healthcare as follows: 1) efficacy, meaning the ability to care or improve health; 2) effectiveness, meaning the degree to which attainable health improvement are realized; 3) efficiency, meaning the ability to obtain the greatest health improvement at the lowest cost; 4) optimality, meaning obtaining the most advantageous balancing of cost and benefits; 5) acceptability, meaning conformity to patient preferences regarding accessibility, patient-doctor relationship, amenities, effect of care, and cost of care; 6) legitimacy, meaning conformity to social preferences concerning all of the above; and 7) equity, meaning fairness in the distribution of care and its effects on health (Wikipedia 2020, para. 1).

According to an article titled "Evaluating the Quality of Medical Care: Donabedian's Classic Article 50 Years Later," Berwick and Fox (2016) analyzed and quoted some of the Donabedian's philosophical thoughts that "systems . . . are enabling mechanisms only. It is the ethical dimension of individuals that is essential to a system's success . . . the secret of quality is love. You have to love your patient, you have to love your profession, you have to love God" (Wikipedia 2020, para.2).

Chapter 4

Nursing Homes in the
Historical Perspective

It is often said that in life's journey, knowing where you came from does not only determine where you are going, it may also help shape the rest of your journey and your successful arrival at your destination. There is also a look-back period in which there is an assessment to determine any changes that could have been made or need to be made to ensure a better future. The journey the nursing home industry has made, commonly known as starting with the almshouse, is no exception. This chapter is important because there is a general belief that in human endeavor, knowing the past can help control or shape the future, and the ability to look back determines what improvement has occurred.

The concept of almshouses dating back to tenth-century Britain is oftentimes considered as the mother of today's nursing homes in the United States and elsewhere. In medieval Britain, almshouses were established to "provide a place of residence for poor, old and distressed people" (Wikipedia 2017, para.1). Almshouses, which is the English name for the same institution as the poorhouses of the United States, were "tax-supported residential institutions to which people were required to go if they could not support themselves" (Crannell, 2000).

The concept of almshouses was brought over to the United States in the early 1600s by the English settlers when this "English tradition of almshouse was introduced to the Commonwealth of Pennsylvania by its founder, William Penn. The Maryland legislature created almshouses in Anne Arundel County, financed by property taxes on landowners throughout the state. Massachusetts also had a long tradition of almshouses" (Wikipedia 2017, para 1). The intention of developing these institutions was to have a place for the poor, elderly, disabled, and other folks who were unable to live independently.

In the beginning, there were laws called the Poor Laws, which were administered by Overseers of the Poor (Wagner, 2005). Authorities who were assigned this duty were usually chosen from those who were well-to-do or wealthy, and who had no experience with poverty. The distribution of aid was not equal for those who needed it. Rather, aid depended upon matters such as the person's financial standing in the community, the length of time lived in the town, the social status of the person, and the reason for the need of help. Those who were lucky enough to receive aid saw it, possibly, in the form of food or fuel. The goal of the authorities was to move those they labeled as undeserving of help, such as men whom they thought should be able to work and women considered to be sexually immoral, into the almshouses and poorhouses of the particular town (Wagner, 2005). Care in these establishments was hit and miss; some residents received care, but most did not.

Conditions Encountered in Almshouses and Poorhouses

According to an investigation carried out by Dr. C. William Chancellor for the State Board of Health of Maryland in 1877 ("Almshouse Care," 2004), the living conditions and care of the patients in almshouses was deplorable. After conducting a thorough inspection (2004), he commented that, "For the insane, there is written over the portal of the almshouse as those over the infernal regions, 'Whoever enters here leaves hope behind'" ("Almshouse Care," para. 1).

Patients did not have beds, but filthy blankets and pillows on the floor in rows, with the toes of one person touching the head of the next. Those who were considered mentally insane were kept full-time in restraints without adequate bedding or nutrition. Eventually, almshouses were designated as holding and living spaces for the mentally insane. The African-American insane were treated worse than the local farm animals, with no indoor plumbing, daily hygiene, or cleansing of the incontinent; and there was, often, an "almshouse odor" ("Almshouse Care," para. 4) that was encountered upon entering any of the buildings. While restraints of patients had been denounced by most medical professionals, the attendants, who were sometimes local farmers, had no training, and would consistently keep the patients in restraints. There was at least one patient who was reported of dying from being in restraints when he developed gangrene in both hands. Considering the conditions these patients endured, most did not make it out with their lives ("Almshouse Care," 2004).

The conditions were much poorer for African-Americans than those of white patients, where they were housed in overcrowded, unclean slaves' quarters. For most counties in Maryland, it was illegal to house white and black patients together; however, some counties violated these laws and allowed cohabitation ("Almshouse Care," 2004).

African-Americans and the mentally insane were not the only lower-class people abused and mistreated in the almshouses. Because of misappropriation of funds, insufficient quantity of poor taxes, and an ever-increasing number of poor and indigent persons, there was never enough money to take care of the things that the needy required to survive. As a result, in Philadelphia, the authorities began indenturing children and young adults to those members who were able to pay, and in return, they agreed to teach and educate them with valuable skills that they could then use to be productive members of society once released. Due to the indiscretion and dishonesty of many of those involved, children were forced from their families, sent far from their homes, and used as free labor. No family or child was immune to this, and it was a great fear of parents that their children would be taken from them, never to see them again (Kaktins, 2016).

Over time, the types of patients that were admitted to almshouses changed. Those who were mentally ill, physically disabled, unemployed men, and women who were considered to be immoral or prostitutes were removed, and almshouses became a refuge for the elderly. Because of this, the almshouse became a place where the elderly were sent to die, and they were greatly feared by all. According to Wagner (2005), a ballad was written during this time by Will Carleton. He penned "Over the Hill to the Poorhouse," which intimately portrays the position the elderly were in:

> *Over the hill to the poor-house I'm trudgin' my weary way. I a woman of 70 and only a trifle gray. I, who am smart an' chipper, for all the years I've told, as many another woman that's only half as old. What is the use of heapin' on me a pauper's shame? Am I lazy or crazy? Am I blind or lame? True, I am not so supple, nor yet so awful stout: But charity ain't no favor. If one can live without over the hill to the poorhouse—my childr'n dear, goodbye! Many a night I've watched you when only God was nigh: And God'll judge between us; but I will always pray that you shall never suffer the half I do today (Carleton, 1882).*

The Development of Medical Education in Modern Hospitals and Nursing Homes

Before the early 1900s, the medical care administered to those confined to almshouses and poorhouses was negligible for those living there. In Richmond, Virginia, a plea for the introduction of skilled nurses in all almshouses was made by Reverend Caroline Bartlett Crane in 1908 (Dock, 1908). A table demonstrated in this article shows the number of nurses practicing between the years 1880–1905 increased from 157 to 5,795. The number of hospital beds also increased during the years between 1900 and 1905 from 84,227 to 145,506 (Dock, 1908). This was the beginning of the responsibilities of the modern hospitals, nursing homes, and hospices.

As the nineteenth century eased into the twentieth century, major medical discoveries and accomplishments, as well as the introduction of medical education for physicians and nurses, helped bring about accessible healthcare to those previously housed in almshouses (Gourevitch, Malaspina, Weitzman, and Goldfrank, 2008). Some would also argue that it was the increased demand for change alongside criticism of the nineteenth century that signaled the beginning of the demand for quality in healthcare services, including nursing homes.

In the nineteenth century, John Morgan proposed that in order to obtain a medical degree, an apprenticeship of three to four years and at least two terms of two to three months each be completed at a medical school. Even though hundreds of medical schools opened during this time, most were in it for the profits and not the excellence of education. Many people who were completely incompetent and incapable of becoming physicians were admitted into these programs, and as a result, doctors were produced who were totally unfit to become upstanding physicians and fulfill their profession.

The president of the New York Medical Society (1988) stated that "with few exceptions, practitioners are ignorant, degraded, and contemptible" (Bloch, p. 230). Another statement was made by the chairman of the recently formed AMA (1988), "The profession, once venerated, has become corrupt and degenerate. Many are unworthy of the Association by intellectual culture or moral discipline" (Bloch, p. 230). Because of such destitution in the field of medicine, most people feared going to the doctor, and relied on natural and home remedies to cure their ailments. Even though medicine was in a grim state during this time, amazing discoveries were made, such as the difference in the causes of typhus and typhoid, hydrochloric acid in the stomach, the use of anesthesia such as ether in surgical procedures, and the isolation of adrenaline (Bloch, 1988).

Chapter 5

Holistic Management and the Imperative of Change in Nursing Homes. Are We Ready?

This chapter deals with the reality of change and the imperative for nursing homes to improve nursing home quality. The demand for change in nursing homes is based on its early institutional neglect and the recognition that the elderly in our societies deserve a dignified standard of living in their waning years.

What is the meaning of change, and what type of change does the nursing home industry need? In general, change means different things to different people in different situations. Causes and effects of change are different as well, but it is noteworthy that in all walks of life, including nursing homes, change is real and always forthcoming. "Men and women are faced with new situations to which they must respond. These situations reflect such factors as the introduction of new techniques, new ways of making a living, changes in place of residence, innovations in ideas and social values" (Merrill, 1961, 332).

In the main, change can be a natural or man-made occurrence that forces humans to readjust, adapt to, or rethink new positions in life in order to survive well. In recent years, the one area of change that is publicly felt and discussed, with the public demanding urgent action to reverse its causes and effects on human environment, is climate change. But climate change is not the only change occurring in our human ecology. There are other types of change taking place around us at different rates and intensities. The intensity of change can be described as change in which its onset is so acutely felt negatively or positively that it requires an immediate human action.

The event of 9/11 in the United States represented causation of change that required immediate action to improve the nation's national security, especially at the airports and for air travel in general. The automobile industry's decision to update models of cars has used the concept of change to incentivize consumers to buy new cars. The Industrial Revolution of the 1760s marked the transition from primitive to modern mechanized manufacturing, agricultural, transportation, and communication systems, and is credited for the improved standard of living in the goods and services mankind enjoys today.

In a book titled *To Have or To Be?*, Fromm (1976, xi) wrote:

> *Man has entered a new era of evolutionary history, one in which rapid change is a dominant consequence. He is contending with a fundamental change, since he has intervened in the evolutionary process. He must now better appreciate this fact and then develop the wisdom to direct the process toward his fulfillment rather than toward his destruction.*

More succinctly, Kneller (1971, 77), in his book titled *The Foundations of Education*, explained the concept of change as a developmental process, and wrote:

> *A person changes because his needs at one stage of his development cannot be met by the behaviors that were adequate at an earlier stage. At the point where society attaches certain values and attitudes to specific developmental stages, change becomes a matter of developing new strategies to meet new demands and expectations*

Whether change occurs imperceptibly or with a bang, it is needful to research it and adjust to it. Socrates (470–399 BC) is quoted as maintaining: the secret of change is to focus all of your energy, not on fighting the old but building the new. In all forms of human endeavors, the opposite of change is stagnation, which is in contrast to human nature. Scientists in different fields tend to agree on the inevitability of change in our personal lives, businesses, in science and technology. There are differences in opinion, however, on the variabilities of human reaction to change, falling within the continuum of either embracing change, fearing change, avoiding change, fighting change, anticipating change, or initiating change.

Change being an actualized and unavoidable event in our lives, big or small, cannot be escaped or ignored. It is our view also that it is better to embrace change than fight it, and to initiate change that anticipates good fortune. The idea of initiating change is to improve the quality of human lives, which is embodied in the goodwill of the change agent. And like Thomas Edison (1847–1931), there is that belief that even if change fails, there is always a value-added effect in the lessons learned in the process of perfecting the future.

Providers of care and administrators in nursing homes are reminded of this prospect of change. Accordingly, Gordon and Stryker (1983, 82) echoed the necessity of change in the management of nursing homes due to the complexities and challenges of managing a social- and medical-oriented organization. With specific emphasis on administrators' function, they stated "as administrator of a nursing home today, you are managing a constantly changing organization which never retains the status quo for any length of time." This means acquiring the ability not only to embrace something new, but to develop specific management skills of adapting to a different and unforeseen circumstance associated with new situations.

Change circumstances, like adopting a holistic view in nursing home management, may require shifting things around, changing peoples' minds, or reaching for new ideas. In a book titled *Teaching and Learning in Adult Education*, Miller (1964, 158) quoted John Dewey as emphasizing "the need for skill in problem-solving as the most effective method of dealing with the introduction of change." Additionally, Miller, favoring group participation and decision-making, suggested that "solutions which a group of affected individuals reach may not be the most efficient solutions to the problem, but they are almost bound to be the most acceptable ones and consequently the only workable ones" (158). It is within this body of thought that nursing home administrators, as part of their job description, are change agents who must be able to motivate and inspire confidence in the members of their group to bring about change for the sake of improving nursing home quality.

Semantically, the act of change goes hand in hand with the act of overhauling or reforming something, most especially if the expected outcome had not been realized. It goes without saying that the definition of insanity is doing something the same way over and over again but expecting different results (Einstein, 1879–1955). In nursing homes, the word *reform* has been popularly used, as in the Nursing Home Reform Act (NHRA) of 1987, with its biggest achievement being the establishment of the minimum data set (MDS), standardizing nursing home care throughout the United States. MDS assessments are designed not only to help nursing home staff identify each resident's health needs and standardize the billing process, but also recognize the resident's bill of rights. The first two reasons demand that a resident's assessments be accurate and holistic, with every effort made to avoid "garbage in, garbage out," and the third reason is a reminder to treat residents with respect and dignity in an environment that promotes love and affection.

Historically, the NHRA became a part of OBRA '87 as initiated by the Institute of Medicine in 1986. As we have documented elsewhere, OBRA '87's regulatory reform since its inception has been incremental and less radical, leaving the negative public opinion, attitudes, and behavior about nursing home care unchanged. A review titled "Update on the Public's Views of Nursing Homes and Long-Term Care Services" on the achievement of NHRA and OBRA '87 was conducted in 2007 after twenty years of implementation. This survey found that "there are still concerns about the progress that has been achieved since this legislation and the overall quality of long-term care" (Wikipedia 2019 para 1).

In an article titled "Transforming Nursing Home Care," Ersek (2015, 1) stated that "there is widespread fear about nursing home care, which in many cases is warranted." Commenting on "Nursing Home Quality: Continued Improvements Needed in CMS's Data and Oversight," Dickson (2018, 1) stated "we testified that CMS's data showed mixed results—they showed an increase in consumer complaints along with improvements in the quality of care."

Goldsmith (1993, xxv) saw nursing homes as organizations needing transitional updates and adjustments in response to the needs of the individuals who inhabit them, and predicted that "no longer are nursing homes merely residences for frail elderly, but rather they are in the process of becoming an exceedingly interesting amalgam of both social services oriented organizations and technologically sophisticated clinical facilities."

A true change that is waiting to be realized in nursing home care is envisioned not to comprise of legislations alone, but the ability of care providers (entrepreneurs) to manage all aspects of nursing homes holistically, and not as an organization with an unintegrated fission of technological, clinical, managerial abilities and skills. It is also important that nursing homes are viewed as unique organizations where the measurement of success would only lie in the quality of service as perceived by the residents, their families, and advocates.

Unlike in other business organizations, public opinion about nursing home care is very consequential, emotional, and powerful. By its own nature, it is the service satisfaction that the residents, families, and advocates see and feel that should be seen as the overriding factor in the shareholders' positive return on investment. In many aspects of our socioeconomic lives, it is the public opinion in general that has been noted to induce change. In nursing homes, it is the allegations of abuse and neglect of vulnerable residents that has reminded the lawmakers and the public of the stories of almshouses/poorhouses that generate their call for change.

In many aspects of our business or personal life, at one time or another, change is expected. Whenever change occurs, it can be abruptly, imperceptibly, or gradually felt. Either way, change requires much of our attention to ensure necessary planning in areas needing behavioral, financial, or environmental adjustment. In general, it must be noted that "while all changes do not lead to improvement, all improvement requires change. The ability to develop, test, and implement changes is essential for any individual, group, or organization that wants to continuously improve" (Wikipedia, 2017, para. 1).

Change, in health care in general and in nursing homes in particular, being essential, has been seen to be gradual, if not imperceptible.

Nevertheless, researchers whose interests are in nursing homes would agree that in America, 1935 was a year of change in the industry's growth and development, paving the way for further legislations targeting quality of care; quality of life of residents in public housing; research in medicine, education, technology; and general interest in the field of gerontology.

When we say that change in the nursing home industry has been gradual and imperceptible, we are comparing it to other industries like the automobile industry, in which change can be readily noticed. The picture shows a 1935 Chevy Sedan dating back to the same year that the Social Security Act was passed and the 2017 dramatizes a noticeable change. Change in nursing homes can be expected to follow a similar pattern, requiring entrepreneurial and governmental commitments to make a nursing home a home away from home, understanding its complexities and current perceptions.

The need for change and improvement in caring for America's elderly and disabled in nursing homes is becoming more and more evident as the numbers of the infirm are steadily increasing. President Franklin D. Roosevelt provided the first step by instituting the Social Security and Old Age Assistance Act in 1935, as well President B. Johnson, who signed the Medicaid program into law, intended to eliminate the concept of almshouses and poorhouses and give the indigent population a decent livelihood, paving the way for for-profit or not-for-profit organizations to get involved in nursing home as a business.

But it seems that from 1930 to 1960 the United States did not see the development of modern nursing homes that meet needs of the so-called poor people as important, or had taken baby steps toward it. The fact that it took over 300 years (1600–1935) for the government to try to intervene in correcting the condition in almshouses/poorhouses and another thirty years (1935–1965) for the Medicaid program to be enacted has propped the perception of today's nursing homes to remain negative for so long.

There tends to be a lingering memory of what happened in almshouses, the qualification and types of people who resided there. They were poor, destitute, and were treated as such. To an extent that nursing homes today are institutions for poor people and thereby comparable to almshouses can be justifiable, but the irony is the feeling of an individual's self-esteem and self-worthiness associated with poverty. Medicaid, which pays for the majority of nursing home residency, is a poverty-based program. Most people who enter nursing homes have to meet a certain Medicaid poverty requirement based on their income level. However, those individuals with declined activities of daily living (ADLs) and health conditions who need nursing home placement but have high income would be required to spend down.

We also see the negative perception of nursing homes from the perspective of ageism. The self-hatred stemming from our inability to accept aging as a normal process of life has an effect of generating hatred for self and toward others. In societies where the glamour of youthfulness is more celebrated than the wisdom of the aged, and poverty is negatively stereotyped, nursing homes tend to become a fertile ground for negativity, demanding a psychosocial change to value human life in its totality, from cradle to grave.

Cultivating a sense of self-value and being valued is needed as part of quality care in nursing homes. To dramatize this point, Cox (1989) wrote:

> *Older people think of themselves as being much younger than they are. One researcher asked a group of elderly people to describe themselves, and a woman in her 80s brought out a picture of herself taken 40 years earlier. When asked if she had a more recent photo, she reluctantly handed over one taken the year before, protesting, "It's terrible. It's not me at all."*

There is the frequent comparison of nursing homes to acute care hospitals, but before this comparison can be completely valid, there must first be an understanding of the disease process of the aged and the distinction in the difficulty of everyday life of caring for people with acute health issues versus those with chronic health problems that are associated with aging within the concept of institutionalization. Currently, nursing homes are more susceptible to having negative reviews than acute hospitals. Frequently cited preventable or unpreventable characteristics of nursing homes as causes of nursing home negative reviews relate to family conflicts, food taste, urine smells, resident lack of privacy, resident abuse and neglect by staff, resident to resident inappropriate interactions, wandering residents, noise, and low expectation of residents surviving well after admission, to name a few. Forbes (2017) has accessed this controversy and wrote:

> *Seniors often resist living in a nursing home as there are many taboos that surround them. For example, in the old days people would send their parents to nursing homes and they would die. So, people begin thinking that nursing homes were a place to die. This is certainly not true. Nursing homes nowadays are places where seniors can thrive and live happy lives*

We expect the reluctance to accept nursing homes as an ideal alternative place for the aged, the sick, and infirm to linger on for a while, as most of the resistance dwells in human psychology of conscience and poverty, change, and culture. McCullough and Wilson (1995, 201–203), in their analysis of the problem, wrote:

> *In nursing homes and rehabilitation centers, many of the most vexing ethical problems have to do not with the big ticket of life and death dilemmas, but rather with the small-scale conflicts of everyday life . . . residents of nursing homes and other long-term care facilities actually live and cohabit in these institutions. In these home-like spaces, each resident's desires, interests, and actions can impact directly on the interests and legitimate expectations of others. Patients who wander into others' rooms, make loud noises, or refuse to bathe have a direct impact on the quality of life of other residents and the staff.*

These long-term facilities do not only include solely nursing homes, which are also referred to as skilled nursing facilities, but also assisted-living facilities and continuing-care retirement communities. Nursing homes, where approximately 70 percent of America's elderly reside, provide skilled nursing care for both acute and chronic conditions, as well as therapy assisting in activities of daily living.

Assisted-living facilities are much less hospital-like and allow patients to maintain some of their freedoms while having the extra medical and safety support they would not get at home. With the development of assisted-living facilities, the numbers of elderly being admitted to nursing homes has decreased. In a report produced by the American Association of Homes and Services for the Aging, approximately 900,000 Americans live in assisted-living facilities (Nochomovitz). Continuing-care retirement communities consist of a skilled nursing facility, but the care that the patients receives is based on their individual care requirements.

Lastly, patients may choose to have their care take place in their homes, with family members providing support as well as home health services, such as hospice. Patients who are able to remain in their homes also have the added benefit of not being exposed to the infectious diseases seen in skilled facilities.

Nursing homes (skilled facilities) today still carry the fear and hopelessness of a person living out their final days in an institution. While the care is a far cry from what was experienced in almshouses, the professionalism among many of the staff is lacking, and abuse of patients still occurs, even with the increasing amount of education required to work in these institutions. There are also, on the other end of the spectrum, many nurses, aides, and technicians who are dedicated in their work and make the lives of the patients better when these people may have no other human contact other than the nurses and staff. While there are still many challenges, there are also opportunities for change in the management approach in nursing homes that ensure improvement in nursing home quality. Consequently, the holistic management approach is introduced to give managers of nursing homes a different and better perspective than afforded in the traditional management approach.

For example, we believe that managers who train themselves to see the whole organizational picture in order to manage the complexities inherent in the nursing home operation and in each resident are not only the managers of the future for nursing homes, but also the change agents to bring improvement and sustainability in nursing home quality.

In a study titled "Effective Factors in Providing Holistic Care: A Qualitative Study," Zamanzadeh et al. (2015), referencing nursing functions, wrote:

> Holistic care is a comprehensive model of care. Most previous studies have shown that most nurses do not apply this method. Examining the effective factors in nurses' provision of holistic care can help with enhancing it. Studying these factors from the point of view of nurses will generate real and meaningful concepts and can help to extend this method of caring . . . Establishing appropriate educational, management systems, and promoting religiousness and encouragement will induce nurses to provide holistic care and ultimately improve the quality of their caring (Wikipedia 2020, para. 1).

Impact of Government Involvement in Nursing Homes: Funding, Regulations, and Licensing

One of the reasons for government involvement in nursing homes in the United States was to address what was perceived as poor living and health conditions in these institutions. Throughout their history, starting from almshouses, nursing homes and long-term care facilities have not been known for their cleanliness and infection control measures, or their excellence in medical care and the compassion of the people who worked there, from the cleaning staff to nurses and physicians. Therefore, for a long time, these institutions have failed to win the public respect they rightly deserve. But long-term care for the elderly is currently evolving into areas that are more desirable and appropriate to the individual's needs. They are continuously required to show components of the system that demonstrate quality. While changes have been made to improve quality in these institutions, again, they are evolving. More actions still need to take place to ensure that the individuals who are living and being cared for receive the best possible treatments available.

In their commentary on nursing home quality, its history and its measurements, Castle and Ferguson (2010) discuss monitoring methods (Castle & Ferguson, 2010). In defining quality, there are many different definitions that can be considered, but many are generalized and can be problematic and subjective, failing to fully realize their value for the nursing home system. Quality indicators riddle the language rather than quality measures, and the authors note that the "approach of Donabedian is valuable" (Castle and Ferguson, 2010), who proposed that measurements of quality can be measured through processes, structures, and outcomes. Process and outcomes help determine whether or not things done to or for a patient are desirable or not, and structural measures are related to the organization itself (Castle and Ferguson, 2010).

In the late 1960s, certification by the newly designed government Medicaid and Medicare programs was essential in order for the nursing homes to receive reimbursement for patients covered under these programs. The Health Care Financing Administration (HCFA) was founded in 1977, specifically to develop and form standards for this certification process. However, with each passing year, the medical and care requirements of each patient became increasingly more complex (Castle and Ferguson, 2010). New committees and reporting agencies were formed, such as the IOM and GAO reports, which focused on numerous factors found during inspections. The Nursing Home Reform Act was instituted in 1987 with forty-seven changes that were recommended for all nursing homes, but not all of these were placed into effect until 1995 (Castle and Ferguson, 2010).

While numerous changes have been made over the entire course of nursing home history, with many different intentions and results, the progress has been slow and tedious. Even with the creation of indicators and measures, there is no one single factor (or a global measure) that can be tested or instituted to rate the quality of each individual nursing home and the entire system as a whole (Castle and Ferguson, 2010).

There are many areas that will continue to have to be addressed and assessed with the implementation of rules and regulations concerning things such as licensure and certification, more stringent requirements for employees working in these homes, and an increase in the amount of education that nurses and physicians need to obtain to care for the patients. As we move ahead in medical care for the elderly, there needs to be a system set in place that they can eventually trust (and their families also) to have their complete medical and psychiatric care in their best interests.

Nursing homes, as we know them today, have gone through tremendous changes throughout their long and complicated history, beginning with almshouses and ending with the culmination of present-day nursing homes and assisted-living facilities. With the inception of almshouses and poorhouses, the population consisted mostly of the elderly whose family members were unable to care for them due to being forced out of work by the Industrial Revolution and wartime. By the nineteenth century, almshouses were occupied by not only the elderly but also the mentally ill, the disabled, and orphans. These institutions were known for their debasement and humiliation of the unfortunate souls in their care.

In 1935, the federal government of the United States, for the first time since the conception of almshouses, engaged in an attempt to annihilate these abominable homes by allotting pensions through the Social Security Act to the needy elderly as long as they were not institutionalized (Crannell, 2000). This was an attempt to enable them to become financially independent and live on their own. However, those involved in the creation of the Social Security Act as a way to relieve the burden of the almshouses misinterpreted the magnitude of the number of patients who were there for physical disabilities, mental illness, and illnesses that required medical and nursing care that could not be provided at the level of the household. The government was determined to decimate the sordid almshouses, and in acknowledgment of the failure of providing the needy elderly with a pension, all patients residing in almshouses were denied money from the government. This meant that those who could not live on their own due to physical or mental ailments had to depend on private institutions for their care.

The government, shrewdly, at this point, turned all public institutions into private establishments, and therefore, the money the patients received from their pensions was siphoned into the finances of each. Through the elimination of the almshouses, the modern nursing home and assisted-living institutions were created.

By taking a look at the lengthy history of nursing homes as they are known today, this chapter will afford a better understanding of the development of the institutions and the lives of not only the patients but also the employees, including physicians and nurses.

According to an article titled "Long-Term Care in the United States: A Timeline," from 1935 to 2015, there have been twenty-six documented legislations and their timelines by the lawmakers in the United States Congress that have impacted the conduct of operation of nursing homes to improve the quality of lives in nursing homes. In the article, it is stated that:

> *Long-term care (LTC) in the United States has evolved over the course of the last century to better serve the needs of seniors and persons with disabilities. This timeline outlines the major milestones in LTC from the nursing home era, which created an institutional bias in LTC, to the era of home and community based services (HCBS) and integration, and into the era of health reform and beyond. These milestones include key legislation and court decisions that were instrumental in providing LTC funding; improving the quality of care and safety in nursing homes; and allowing people with LTC needs to stay in their communities. Despite these successes, proposals by commissions and legislators for broader and more comprehensive national LTC policies have not been fully realized; though efforts in this area continue (Wikipedia 2017, para. 1).*

The 1935 Social Security Act (SSA), which only allowed payments to be made directly to poor individuals, not to institutions, was reversed in 1950, allowing payments for medical care to be made directly to institutions and not to beneficiaries. The Civil Rights Act of 1964, which was initiated by President John F. Kennedy before his assassination and signed into law by President Lyndon B. Johnson, was designed to prohibit discrimination in employment, public housing, and institutions such as nursing homes. This legislation, which outlawed all forms of discrimination based on race, color, religion, sex, or national origin, has been known as an important landmark legislation for not only allowing nursing homes to manage today's diverse nursing home population but to assure all residents equal treatment and mental and physical protection based on individual rights and freedoms guaranteed in the United States Constitution and the Bill of Rights.

Cumulatively, the 1776 Declaration of Independence statement by Thomas Jefferson that "all men were created equal," the 1791 Bill of Rights written by James Madison for the "protection of individual liberties," and the Civil Rights Law of 1964 signed by Lyndon B. Johnson outlawing discrimination based on "race, color, religion, sex, or national origin" are platforms for what is now known in today's nursing homes as the "resident quality of life" regulation. Notable also is the 1965 Medicare and Medicaid Act signed into law by President Lyndon B. Johnson, which has made the federal government of the United States the biggest payer source for nursing homes.

In 1953, the Department of Health, Education, and Welfare (HEW), which was already formed, was to protect the health of citizens and provide essential human services, but its impact on nursing homes was not felt until between 1977 and 1980. It was in 1980 that the former HEW became the current Department of Health and Human Services (HHS) as an overseer of the Health Care Financing Administration (HCFA), currently renamed as the Center for Medicare& Medicaid Services (CMS). It has a wide range of responsibility over nursing homes, including the Office of Inspector General, which investigates and prosecutes nursing home criminal cases. It must be noted that as a result of reported rampant fraud and abuse in nursing homes, an additional amendment to the SSA was necessitated in 1967, which authorized statutory involvement by state governments to oversee nursing home operations and to license and supervise nursing home administrators. Accordingly, state governments in the United States were on their way to developing state laws and other indigenous modalities to supervise all nursing homes participating in Medicaid and Medicare program.

Today, Medicaid and Social Security benefits continue to pay for nonskilled residents in nursing homes while Medicare pays for the skilled care that may arise. Even though the funding sources and oversight provisions backed by laws and statutes for nursing homes were fully established by 1967, there were no meaningful performance standards set by any regulatory agency. Unlike the acute care hospital, which Congress had mandated its accreditation and supervision to the Joint Commission on Accreditation of Healthcare Organization (JACHO), the nursing home industry chartered a different path of development. Hence, the problem of measuring quality of care and other operational outcomes in nursing homes remained problematic for the government throughout the periods of the 1950s, 1960s, 1970s, and early parts of the 1980s. But with CMS takeover, the Omnibus Budget Reconciliation Act (OBRA) was enacted in 1987, with provisions that began to shape nursing homes toward better care outcomes, and away from the syndrome of the almshouse.

In an article titled "Nursing Home Regulation: History and Expectation," Morford (2017) wrote, "Finally, the results of these changes are projected in terms of new outcome-oriented requirements and a broad range of new enforcement authorities." Accordingly, OBRA had two major accomplishments; namely, setting up the requirements that nursing homes must meet for continual participation in the Medicare and Medicaid program, and establishing the enforcement requirements in which state agencies were assigned the responsibility of conducting periodic oversight supervision and inspections to determine compliance, as contained in the Code of Federal Regulations 1987a, 1987b and 1987c.

During this transitional period of the 1980s, individual states were also crafting their own nursing home laws. State laws were tailored to meet the health and administrative needs of that specific state that were not in conflict with federal health laws or the constitution of the United States. Specifically, it is within the context of these federal and state laws that the role, requirements, responsibilities, accountability, and leadership of the nursing home administrator and that of the governing body, as indicated, have become crucially important. According to OBRA's mandated regulation CFR 483.75 (F490-F522), they must apply sufficient resources, adopt management and leadership styles that are more responsive to the demands associated with managing the nursing home successfully, and states "the facility must be administered in the manner that enables it to use its resources effectively and efficiently to attain or maintain the highest practicable physical, mental, and psychosocial well-being of each resident" (Pate and Yale 2009, 353).

The Impact of Baby Boomers, Cultural Diversity, and Holistic Management in Nursing Homes

The United States of America was born as a multicultural, multiracial, and multiethnic society. For many years, it operated under racial and ethnic segregation, inequality, and brutality of one race over others. Schools, churches, and nursing homes were segregated. Neighborhoods were segregated into white, black, China towns, and Indian reservations, impacting health care and social interactions among citizens. Racial and ethnic segregation practice in the United States also brought with it social instability, violence, nonviolent resistance, and knowledge of civil disobedience. The baby boomer generation was born to inherit these social evils and injustices, as well as to become the generation not only to resist it but also to reimagine new social norms of freedom and equality.

Like the rest of society, nursing homes were not immune to the multitude of societal challenges for which change was needed. However, within the concept of racial segregation, nursing homes continued to operate safely in their segregated neighborhoods. Today, despite racial and ethnic desegregation laws, there still exist pockets of predominately white or black nursing homes.

In 1866, a Civil Right Act was signed, recognizing the citizenship of all males born in the United States. And in 1964, a Civil Right Act was signed, prohibiting discrimination in public accommodations and federally funded programs on the basis of race, color, religion, sex, or national origin. However, interracial marriages and cohabitation remained illegal for fifty-three years, which was resolved in the 1967 Supreme Court case involving the marriage of Richard and Mildred Loving.

A high number of baby boomer retirees are expected to enter these residential facilities, and the impact of the civil right laws, civil right movement, and racial desegregation is likely to be felt, capable of making the baby boomers agents of change in nursing homes. Nursing home operations are federally funded programs through Medicare and Medicaid. Racial desegregation in the United States and racial cohabitation in its institutions are noted for taking gradual steps from 1619 to present. With much more work remaining to be done, managers of human organizations are required to ensure ethno-cultural and racial equanimity.

Healthcare providers and nursing home administrators in particular are expected to be aware of the constitutional, legislative, and regulatory mandates for nondiscriminatory practices. According to health care research, racial desegregation and cohabitation among baby boomers in healthcare institutions like nursing homes will pose social, medical, and clinical challenges for care providers. The baby boomer generation is predicted to have a higher rate of age-related and lifestyle-related social, medical, and clinical issues than their predecessors upon entering nursing homes. In an article titled "Racial and Ethnic Disparities in Social Engagement among US Nursing Home Residents," Li and Cai (2014) wrote that "concerns exist about whether nursing homes can serve appropriately the clinical and psychosocial needs of patients with increasingly diverse ethnic and cultural backgrounds" (Wikipedia 2020, para 2). Similar studies relating to medical and nursing issues have shown no cause for alarm because modern and improved medical and nursing technologies will provide nursing homes the ability to provide residents with quality of care. Nevertheless, it is important to remind nursing home administrators and staffers of the holistic management approach they need to effectively manage residents' quality of life and residents' cohabitation needs in a multicultural, multiracial, yet restrictive institutional setting.

Nursing homes are now admitting residents with different racial and ethnic groups, social class, and lifestyles under one roof, and regulations require them to accommodate residents' lifestyles, independence, individuality, and identity. For care providers who have not yet switched to holistic management and are accustomed to providing institutional one-size-fits-all services, the problem of meeting nursing home quality in the future for residents' personal preferences will increase, not decrease.

Nursing home regulation requires that every resident's historical data that is documented in the intake record must be followed up to ensure that each resident's prior lifestyles and social values continue as much as practicable. Baby boomers who are now living in desegregated nursing homes or are about to enter desegregated nursing homes are likely to bring with them different internalized psychosocial experiences, demanding care providers to be able to provide them with spiritual and psychosocial help as needed, including appropriate admission placements and room-mating.

Every resident's admission should viewed in light of the safety and security of other residents. With the baby boomers entering nursing homes, there is a growing demand to build new types of nursing homes, not only to avoid the present institutional image of nursing homes, unaccustomed to the baby boomers, but to accommodate their demand for privacy and independence. Accordingly, the concept of the Green House and Eden is already taking root, representing the future of nursing homes for the baby boomer generation and beyond.

While holistic care management is recommended at every stage of the residents' nursing home stay, we predict the baby boomers' need for more privacy, food preferences, recreational and psychosocial activities to play a more dominate role in provoking their early maladjustment to their new environment, and the prevalence of resident/resident, resident/staff, or staff/resident aggressions later on. Based on the baby boomers' prior lifestyle, nursing homes must be ready to accommodate their needs for unrestricted freedom of movement, private rooms, demand for personalized fitness programs, sexual freedoms, religious freedoms, illegal drug use, personal computers, personalized laundry service, and a well-stocked library.

The majority of the baby boomers are today's career professionals, who are more likely to require more than BEMS (bingo, eat, medication, and sleep) to keep them satisfied during their residency in nursing homes. In holistic nursing home management, investigating aggressive, inappropriate behaviors involving residents or staff cannot be limited only to search for mental illness, they must also include causations from unfulfilled psychosocial needs of residents and workplace dissatisfaction of staff.

Over the years, human needs theorists like Abraham Maslow, Karen Horney, and others have argued that unmet needs can cause maladaptive behaviors such as anxiety, frustration, aggression, and hostile social interaction in humans. Accordingly, given the amount of human-to-human interaction involved in caregiving in nursing homes, OBRA '87.10(F165–F166) is a mandate that nursing homes must have plans to prevent aggressive and inappropriate behaviors from occurring in their organizations, and must resolve all grievous situations within a reasonable time. In most states, nursing homes are allowed up to thirty days to complete their investigations on accidents or incidents of aggression and physical, sexual, or verbal abuse. Reporting residents' incidents and accidents promptly is a requirement under state LTC regulation.

Managing racial, cultural, and ethnic diversity in nursing homes is a requirement stemming from the United States Constitution. Care providers must manage the boomers of all races who must live in the same institution but have different preferences for language/intonation subcultures, food, religion, body language, music and dance, ageism, classism, greetings and salutation, clothing and adornment, rituals, privacy, and noise, to name a few. They will be more likely to resist the restrictive environment, which aptly describes the present nursing home setting.

Even though the new Greenhouse project and the Eden Alternative are on their way up as an alternative competition to the current traditional nursing home setting, their availability to accommodate the population of the baby boomers is uncertain. Most reports show that there are currently 260 greenhouses in twenty-six states in the United States. The closest bet is the Eden Alternative.

In an article titled "The Green House Project: The Next Big Thing in Long-Term Care," Larson (2015) describes it as a project that "focuses on partnering with nursing homes to help them change the culture, environment, and approach to care to create a habitat for human beings rather than facilities for the frail and elderly" (Wikipedia 2020, para 2). The goal of both the Greenhouse concept and the Eden Alternative is to provide the aged, who normally go to traditional nursing homes, with more privacy, independence, and control.

When the Civil Rights Act of 1964 banned discrimination based on race, color, religion, sex, or national origin . . . racial segregation in schools, employment, and public accommodations, nursing homes were no exception. The OBRA '87:483.10 (F151–F177) mandate is derived from the Civil Rights Act of 1964 as a foundation of the long-term care regulation written to protect the self-determination and rights of nursing home residents, correlating with its current emphasis on residents' quality of life.

Based on the boomers' predispositions and aspirations for inquisitiveness, activism for direct social change, and love for personal freedoms, the demand for participatory relationship of mutual respect between care providers and residents will not only increase, it will be the determinant for residents' quality of life.

Baby boomers in nursing homes are expected to be different in that they will be more knowledgeable and vocal about their rights and self-determination. They will not be passive in asking questions and demanding explanations relating to their care, legal rights, company policies, medical and nursing issues, and most importantly, their freedoms to "do things their own way." Because by the time segregation was abolished, the baby boomers in the United States had already developed their self-concept and self-awareness of what it would mean to them to have rights to be treated equally with dignity and respect.

Today, business institutions like nursing homes are adapting in response to the civil rights laws. Treating residents with dignity and respect, ensuring their rights became the cornerstone of nursing home care enshrined in OBRA '87. It is, however, noteworthy that in nursing homes, despite the regulatory requirement for residents' rights, nursing homes must provide a balance between residents' rights and resident safety, which is complicated regarding residents' mental, physical conditions in one hand and their desire for autonomy, independence, and self-determination on the other. Hence, to prevent resident neglect, resident abuse, violation of resident rights, or misinterpreting the goodwill of nursing homes, the state ombudsman, resident guardians, and the AARP (American Association for Retired Persons) have been acting as watchdogs and mediators.

Who are the baby boomers, and what are some of their characteristics that are worthy of care providers' attention in nursing homes? In an article titled "Baby Boomer Trends," they are characterized as "Trendsetters" (Wikipedia 2017, para.1) known to be born between 1946 and 1964. The title *trendsetters* was coined from the increased birth rates in the period after WWII. Because baby boomers are turning sixty-five years or older in great numbers, their retirement is expected to impact many public policies in housing, Medicare/Medicaid, general healthcare, and nursing home policies in particular.

In a book titled "Long-Term Care for the Elderly," Rabin and Stockton (1987, 4) wrote:

It is the aging of the baby boom cohort, who will begin to reach age 65 in about the year 2010, combined with projections of low to moderate future fertility rates, that leads to the confident prediction of a major increase in the elderly population, both in absolute numbers and as a percentage of the total population . . . resulting in as many as over 70 million baby boomer retirees estimated to be in the pipeline.

In an article titled "Boomers in Nursing Homes: Ready or Not, Here They Come," Siberski and Siberski (n. d) wrote, "the baby boomer generation by their sheer numbers has been prodigious . . . presently they are 75 million strong and will overwhelm society's ability to provide adequate care as they age . . . statements from the younger baby boomers, who are currently in their 50s and 60s and voicing their complaints about LTC facilities indicate that such facilities must undergo changes in various areas" (Wikipedia, 2017, para. 1, 7). Another article, titled "Baby Boomer Trends," noted that by 2030 there will be 78 million baby boomers in the United States, of which "54% of the 78 million American Boomers will be women," with stronger economic, social, and political power in their hands (Wikipedia, 2017, para 1).

In an article titled "The 2030 Problem: Caring for Aging Baby Boomers," Knickman and Snell (2002) worried about available economic resources in 2030, and stated that:

> to meet the long-term care needs of Baby Boomers, social and public policy changes must begin soon . . . the 2030 problem involves the challenge of assuring that sufficient resources and an effective service system are available in thirty years, when the elderly population is twice what it is today. Much of this growth will be prompted by the aging of the Baby Boomers, who will be aged 66–84 (Wikipedia 2020, para. 4-5).

While there is no consensus on how many of these baby boomers will actually need nursing home placement at any given time in the continuum of their aging process, it is evident that today's baby boomers, as they age, are more availed than before with more residential care options, ranging from independent living, assisted living, or home care, which are currently becoming more popular than nursing homes. Nappi (2012), in *The Spokesman-Review*, stated that "so much will change for boomers, compared with how their parents and grandparents experienced life after 65. Most boomers will live through a stage of life that stretches 20 to 30 years after retirement age" (Wikipedia 2017, para.7).

Rust (2016), in an article titled "Nursing Home Fade Even as Baby Boomers Age," stated that:

> *As the senior population grows, it's easy to think that nursing homes will be popping up everywhere. In fact, the opposite is true. After booming for much of the late 20th century, the number of the skilled nursing homes in the United States has flat-lined at about 15,000 for more than a decade. By 2021, that figure could shrink by 20 percent (Wikipedia 2017, para. 1).*

According to the article titled "Baby Boomers Will Become Sicker Seniors Than Earlier Generations," the prediction is that "the next generation of senior citizens will be sicker and costlier to the health care system over the next fourteen years than previous generations . . . we are talking about you, baby boomers" (Wikipedia, 2017, para 1). The article goes on to cite an increase of diabetics in the cohort. Yet another article, titled "Baby Boomers Will Transform Health Care as They Age," indicated that "despite a long life expectancy, boomers had higher rates of hypertension, high cholesterol, diabetes and obesity" (Wikipedia 2017, para. 6).

The baby boomer generation in the United States is known to be the product of the social and political events of the 1960s in which their current sociopolitical values, perception of themselves, perception of others and society are molded. Most of the notable events of the 1960s impacting the boomers' beliefs and sociopolitical consciousness relate to their demand for social change, equality, and an end to racial segregation.

Other issues that helped shape the consciousness of the baby boomers would include work-life changes from the era of the Industrial Revolution to the market-based economies; the concept of the middle class; the civil rights movement; the feminist movement; the signing of the Civil Rights Act of 1964; assassinations of President John F. Kennedy, Dr. Martin Luther King Jr., Robert F. Kennedy, and Malcolm X; the Vietnam War (1955–1975), the antiwar movement, and the 1969 Woodstock.

For them it was a time for soul searching for meaning and for redirecting America and the world sociopolitically. Based on what they endured and achieved for the betterment of humanity, most researchers tend to find the baby boomer generation to be more accomplished than the greatest generation before them.

Across the world, many changes were happening during the post WWII period into the baby boomer years. Decolonization of the third world countries and concept of globalization were taking place. One of the decolonization projects was to educate the indigenous citizens by providing them educational opportunities in host countries abroad. A sizeable number of these foreign students who received western education returned home, but most decided to adopt the host countries as citizens or permanent residents, thereby helping to create multicultural and multiethnic societies in the host countries like France, Great Britain, Germany, and the United States of America. It must be noted that some of these host nations were those who also participated or benefited from colonialism, slave trade, slave ownership, and racial segregation.

Another contributing factor to the rise of a multicultural and multiethnic baby boomer generation in the European countries, and particularly in the United States, after WWII was the changing immigration policy initially favoring European and Asian countries against accepting refugees and people from third world countries. Reimers (1981) wrote:

> *Immigrants coming after 1945 were more apt to be refugees and to be of higher skills than before. And the majority were female. From 1945–1965, most European immigrants were from northern and western European countries, but by the 1970s, southern and eastern European nations supplied*

the bulk of European immigrants to America. After 1965, another important shift was apparent: Third World nations replaced Europe as the major sending regions, and by the 1970, the vast majority of America's latest newcomers were from the Third World (Wikipedia 2017, para. 1).

Chapter 6

Interrelationships: Administrator, Federal, State Agencies, and the Governing Board in the Holistic Nursing Home Management Perspective

In real life, we often hear of the cliché of the chicken and the egg relating to which came first, the chicken or the egg. A similar scenario does sometimes exist in the relationship between the NHA and the governing board due to a blurring line separating the possessor of the regulatory authority from the possessor of the legal authority in nursing home operation. To manage a nursing home successfully, the role each entity plays must be clear. Even though OBRA '87 states "the facility must have a governing body, or designated person functioning as a governing body . . . and the governing body appoints the administrator . . ." [42 CFR 483.75(1) (2)], it takes all stakeholders, including the state and federal government agencies, to practically understand in detail why nursing home quality has continued to remain elusive.

An organization such as the nursing home is generally defined as a social system structured and managed to achieve a stated collective goal. Organizational structure implies the designation of employee roles, functions, and relationships that are predetermined and oftentimes arranged hierarchically upward, with relative ranking importance to ensure a smooth business operation, especially in decision-making.

By LTC regulation, the leader in charge of the nursing home operation is the administrator, who must provide the type of leadership and sufficient staff and materials to ensure quality care.

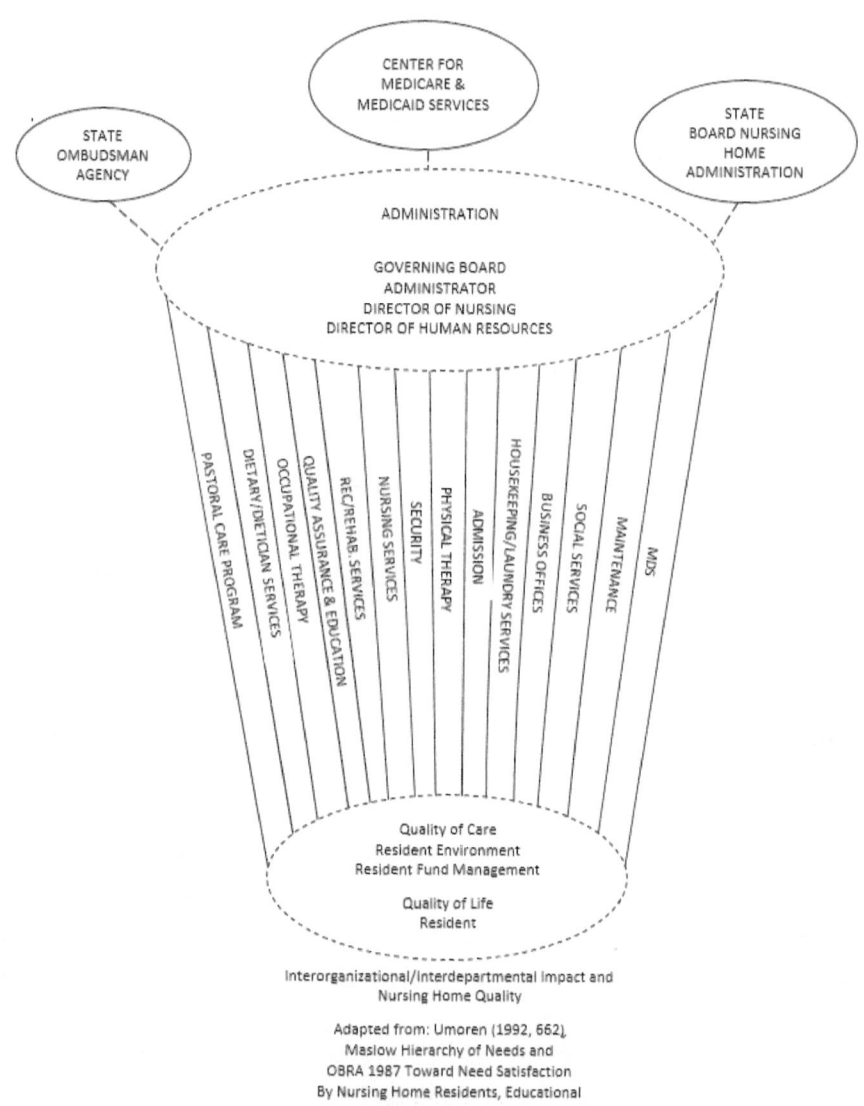

Interorganizational/Interdepartmental Impact and
Nursing Home Quality

Adapted from: Umoren (1992, 662),
Maslow Hierarchy of Needs and
OBRA 1987 Toward Need Satisfaction
By Nursing Home Residents, Educational
Gerontology: An International Journal,

In an article titled "Effective Leadership in Long-Term Care: The Need and the Opportunity," Dana and Olson (n d), in a report presentation to the American College of Health Care Administrators (ACHCA), stated "administrators of nursing homes and a variety of other long-term care settings play a central role in the quality of care and quality of life of the people they serve" (Wikipedia, 2020, para 1). They also observed that "the hectic, unrelenting pace of work along with frequent, unplanned interactions have encouraged and rewarded a crisis management style that makes it difficult for administrators to give priority to leadership process" (Wikipedia,2020, para 5).

In an article titled "Leadership, Staffing and Quality of Care in Nursing Homes," Havig (2011) confirmed that in nursing homes, "leadership and staffing are recognized as important factors for quality of care" (Wikipedia 2020, para 1). Hierarchy of authority assures effective chain of command, communication, and supervision of who does what and when. Usually, in most traditional organizations, there are decision makers and decision takers. In that circumstance, the decision makers ensure that all instructions in the decision are followed even without the involvement of the decision takers in the decision-making process. This is in contrast with the concept of holistic management in which participation in decision-making, communication, collaboration, and interdependence with all organizational members as stakeholders is critical for organizational success.

Covey (1989, 49), in his book titled *The 7 Habits of Highly Effective People*, analyzed the distinction between the concepts of independence, dependence, and interdependence in a group process. Interdependence was corroborated more with an effective group process needed in holistic management, stating "interdependence is a paradigm of we-we can do it; we can cooperate; we can combine our talents and abilities and create something greater, together." For example, as providing sufficient nursing staff in nursing homes tends to reach a road block, isn't it time to apply a collaborative effort between the nursing home industry, the government agencies, and other businesses to join hands for the solution?

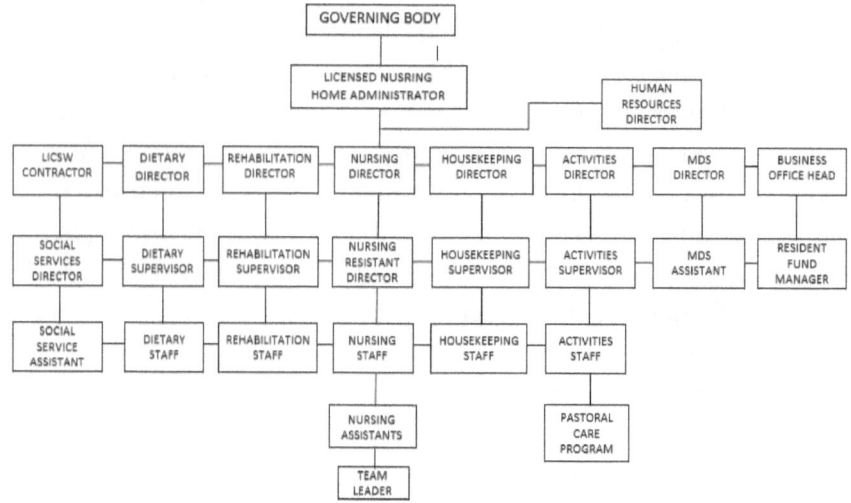

Traditional Organizational Chart, Structure in the
Holistic Nursing Home Management

Meaning of Organizational Chart, Structure, and Holistic Nursing Home Management

All organizational charts are not the same for all organizations, but they form an essential part of every organization's policy and procedures. Organizational charts, in a traditional sense, are developed to represent the road map and the dynamics of each organization. Consistent with holistic management, it shows how all parts within the organization are interconnected. In nursing homes, like in most organizations, the top-down hierarchy of authority—hereby defined as the hierarchy of people with organizational importance, starting with the CEO/chairman to presidents to vice presidents of operations to administrators, on down to departmental directors and rank-and-file employees—can be misleading.

In managing nursing homes, this formal and traditional organizational arrangement that defines the importance of organizational members hierarchically downward has advantages and disadvantages. Creating a holistic organizational chart in response to a preconceived organizational goal, complexity, integration of parts, and evaluative criteria demands leadership, vision, and decision-making.

In holistic management, the organizational chart represents pretty much what the decision maker visualizes the organization to be, who is connected to whom and why, what is connected to what and why, in the organizational system, realizing that every organizational member or station created in the chart must be fully integrated, nurtured, supervised, and functional.

Most of today's organizations, like nursing homes, provide service-oriented work where the majority of the essential functions pertinent to residents' needs are performed by individuals located at lower levels of the organizational chart. It is also noteworthy that most organizational charts are visual aids, shown in diagrams with dotted and solid lines to represent who reports to whom directly or indirectly in the organizational hierarchy. Consequently, there is a tendency to misinterpret staff who have solid lines in the reporting relationships to be more worthy than those represented in the dotted lines.

In holistic management, nothing can be more misleading. We see staff worthiness in relation to their direct contributions to the ultimate goal and objective of the organization. In nursing homes, the goal is to provide services to institutional residents with medical, psycho-physical, and social needs requiring custodial, clinical, or technical skills. Because these essential services are located at the lower levels in the organizational hierarchy, and by the process of absolute importance in the contributions to achieving the organizational collective goal, a question can be raised as to who is more important in the organizational hierarchy.

Implicit also in the holistic nursing home management thinking is the concern in the reward system, which is astronomically tilted in favor of the organizational position an individual holds and not the essentials of work (EOW) one performs in relation to the felt needs of the resident. While we feel comfortable in nagging on the disparity in the reward system between the essentials of work positions and hierarchical management positions, we are not downplaying the difficulty of separating the two, which leaves us with the question: can an organization like the nursing home survive with one without the other? The answer to this question lies in employee motivation and the tough decisions that management in nursing homes must make for the survival of their organizations. It is not uncommon for each organizational member to feel his job position is more important than others. But in nursing homes, we applaud the essentials of work performed by those who provide residents' essential needs, normally requiring the technical skills of certified nursing assistants and other departmental aides.

In holistic management, all organizational members are considered to be important and worthy. But to determine the relative importance of organizational members and establish organizational equity in the employee reward and incentive system, there is a need to consider consequential decisions, task difficulty, and the corresponding damage that can be caused to the organization as a whole if the definition of essentials of work is misplaced.

With regards to the concept of essentials of work in nursing homes, a document from Premier Nursing Academy titled "The Importance of CNAs in Long Term Care" stated that "as a certified nursing assistant . . . you have the most influence on overall patient and family experience, with the ability to create a caring, safe, and home-like environment" (Wikipedia 2020, para 1). Pennington (2003) wrote an article titled "The Role of Certified Nursing Assistants in Nursing Homes," and stated that "CNAs provide 80% to 90% of care to residents in nursing homes . . . their reported turnover rate is as high as 400% in some studies, and the potential pool of CNAs is dwindling" (Wikipedia 2020, para 2). The same research found insufficient staff motivation among the CNAs' cohort in such areas as job enrichment and opportunities, personal growth opportunities, recognition, responsibilities, wages, and a sense of achievement. The importance of holistic management is to assign appropriate recognition to each job function, and to ensure reward equity so that nobody is left behind or forgotten.

When Daniel McCullum (1815–1878) developed the concept of the organizational chart, it coincided with the Industrial Revolution of 1852–1883, and was perceived to be incompatible to holistic management in human organization. It must be noted that the Industrial Revolution was focused on how to mechanize production, which required the organizational chart to provide the structure for the division of labor to ensure manageable parts in organizations. The main criticism of the organizational chart included its failure to take into consideration the importance of the social and interpersonal relationships in human organizations, the organizational flexibility needed with respect to change, and the informal lines of communication needed for an emotional human connection.

The ranking system that is inherent in the concept of the organizational chart was perceived as trending toward an encouragement of human subjugation and was responsible for inequity in workers' reward and incentives. Research also shows that many companies, by failing to update their organizational charts when certain departments close or when employees move from one position to another, rendered the meaning of the organizational chart and structure ineffective. But with the advent of humanistic management involving the work of such clinical and social psychologists and behavior management scientists as Kurt Lewin, Abraham Maslow, Max Wertheimer, B. F. Skinner, Leon Festinger, Douglas McGregor, Victor Vroom, and Frederick Herzberg in managing human organizations, the importance of the organizational chart and structure was redefined consistent with the principles of holistic management.

In an article titled "What is the Right Organizational Structure for the 21st Century?" Levene (2020) wrote:

> *In order for contemporary organizations to thrive, leadership must be willing to critically assess whether their company's structure aligns with its values and goals. This form of big-picture internal assessment often goes unresolved. Changing the tides is hard work. While the hierarchical model enabled industrial-age companies to thrive, the rise of contemporary businesses are facing a new generation of workers who do not want to work in a hierarchy. The flow of knowledge required in successful businesses simply doesn't align with the slow, restrictive style that hierarchies necessitate*

In holistic management, having organizational chart and organizational structure is significant in clarifying and integrating the reporting process of all employees within an organization, defining the decision-making process, creating an information flow from person to person, from one work center to others on how the job is supposed to be done. In an article titled "What is an Organizational Chart?" Bloomenthal (2019) wrote, "an organizational chart is a diagram that visually coveys a company's internal structures by detailing the roles, responsibilities, and relationships between individuals within an entity . . . organizational charts either broadly depict an enterprise company-wide or drill down to a specific department or unit" (Wikipedia 2021, para 1).

The position of a nursing home administrator implying authority, responsibility, accountability, and professional ethics, staff motivation and work assignments are profoundly determined in the company's organizational chart and structures. In nursing home management, the organizational structure shows that an administrator reports directly to the governing board but indirectly to the State Board of Nursing Home Administrators. In the United States, it is the federal government (CMS) in coordination with the state board that mandates that nursing homes must have a governing board or designated persons to function as the governing board.

The governing board is responsible for establishing and implementing policies to assure proper and ethical management of the nursing home. The responsibility of day-to-day operations lie with the administrator and staff as depicted in the organizational chart and structure. The governing board is legally held accountable for any malpractice that may occur in the nursing home. In this regard, the OIG (Office of Inspector General) was established in 2011 in the United States, and charged with criminal and civil enforcement actions against nursing homes for abuse and neglect of residents, including other ethical misconduct. Avoiding fines, civil monetary penalties, and withdrawal from participation in Medicare and Medicaid programs usually give the governing body, the administrator, and staff, within their job function, one more reason to cooperate, to strive for improvement in nursing home quality and ethical standards in nursing homes.

The administrative authority, responsibility, and accountability of the administrator are delegated by the governing board. It requires clarity in the division of labor, decision-making boundary, and a written job description in order to begin the critical relationship that is necessary in forging either a functional or a dysfunctional nursing home. The basic ingredient in a supportive relationship between the governing body and the administrator is trust, collaboration, decision-making, and communication. Trust means a shared belief that the governing body will provide sufficient resources to procure staff and equipment; that the administrator will wisely manage resources and staff without making irreversible mistakes with negative impact on nursing home quality and the investor's bottom line. Collaboration means shared goodwill, concerns, planning, redirection, and decision-making, which flow upward, downward, and across each locus of authority and responsibility within the organizational chart and structure.

Communication means a shared commitment and respect for an effective use of both informal and formal communication lines throughout the nursing home to foster staff morale and productivity. The administrator therefore understands that the top-down delegated authority, responsibility, and accountability given by the governing body must be earned. In much the same vein, the administrator and the governing board must immediately put to use much of the management axiom hypothesizing that managers should not be held accountable for the outcome of the decisions they did not make or fully participate in. There should be an immediate understanding by both the governing board and the administrator that a handed-down decision is contradictory to the principle of holistic management and a rejecting of the concept of a philosopher king.

Chester Bernard (1886–1961) wrote a book titled *The Function of the Executives* and theorized that the three conditions necessary to enhance organizational survival are efficiency, effectiveness, and cooperation. Accordingly, for organizations to be considered efficient, they must satisfy the motives of individuals; for them to be considered effective, they must meet stated organizational goals; and for them to demonstrate a cooperative, there must be shared interests and values.

Bernard viewed "organizations as systems of cooperation of human activities" (Wikipedia 2019, para.4), and by doing so, signaled the acceptance of collaborative, non-unilateral decision-making. Bernard's theory, dating back to 1938, is consistent with the holistic management principles suggesting that those who will be responsible for implementing decisions must sit at the table where those decisions were made.

Nursing home organizations can also benefit from utilizing a delegated authority as long as what is delegated is within the confines of a participatory management. There are certain areas where top-down decision-making is still pervasive in most corporate-oriented nursing homes, requiring scrutiny and research on its effects on nursing home quality.

In the recent decades, all nursing homes have been challenged to maintain high standards in nursing home quality. The nursing home administrator (NHA) has an important position, and the responsibility of meeting nursing home standards of care. Siegel and Zysberg (2016) state that "federal regulations designate the NHA as responsible for facility management, and state-level licensure is a requirement for this position." Licensing of NHAs creates a set of principles and requirements for education, knowledge, and expertise for the position of an NHA, which is a huge professional responsibility. Requirements for licensure as an NHA include passing a national examination, which indicates that entry-level NHAs have possessed specific knowledge, capabilities, skills, and abilities that are crucial to perform competently as an administrator.

NHA requirements vary considerably from state to state as far as formal education and training programs (Siegel and Zysberg). In general however, it must be noted that nursing home administrators are licensed by each state government to ensure that each nursing home operates in the interest of the residents and their families. Importantly, nursing home administrators operate as important go-betweens for the governing board, the state board, or the state ombudsman.

As leaders, they are expected to be able to follow instructions as well as give directions, most especially in the periods of change. Nursing home administrators are oftentimes seen as the persons in charge of the daily management of the nursing home, in which their leadership and managerial acumen is expected. They provide the first contact point in case of any concerns. Even though they are licensed by the State Board of Nursing Home Administrators, who can also revoke their license for cause, it is the governing boards who hire and can fire administrators.

As leaders, nursing home administrators with sufficient training in professional ethics are also often conscious of the need to exercise their autonomy of conscience defined as the right of an individual to refuse to do something requested by another based on conscience, belief, conviction, ethics, or formal training. The question that is seldom asked but requires an answer becomes: Can a nursing home administrator successfully serve two masters without being subservient to one over the other?

This triangulated relationship existing between the licensed nursing home administrator, the governing board, and the state board needs further study. Does the administrator really have a say-so when it comes to major decision-making without producing a conflict of interest between the company's demands and the regulatory demands for nursing home quality? The second question needing an investigation is the impact that the shifting imperative of the administrator's loyalty between the state board and governing board can have on nursing home quality. It is this dual mandate of responsibility, accountability, and loyalty that can sometimes be precarious when most administrators find a variance between regulatory mandates and company policy. Most people would find such conflict inconceivable, since ordinarily it would be the regulatory mandate that would take precedent. Goldsmith (1993, 136), however, has recognized this dilemma between most of the governing boards and administrators, and stated:

> *For the nursing home administrator, the fundamental question is: How can a manager have an effective relationship with a board? At one extreme, the manager must cope with a necessary evil; at the other, the manager is able to utilize the resources that a board can offer. Many managers view their relationship with their board as adversarial*

During the almshouse days and before government funding sources were determined, nursing homes operated as sole proprietary missions for humanitarian purposes to help the poor. There were no financial incentives to operating nursing homes, nor were they considered as profit-making enterprises. But as the demand for more nursing home beds continued, followed by the financial handicap of these sole proprietary missions, government funding became inevitable. The condition for government funding depended on government oversight, comprising of regulations and onsite/offsite inspections. The intention was that when nursing home companies collaborate with government regulations and inspections it would produce nursing home quality. However, in most cases, the so-called government non-interference in the internal day-to-day management of nursing homes was successful in raising the specter of "the behavioristic aspect of capitalistic entrepreneurship" (Umoren 1994, 112).

As the government money was pouring in, the industry was able to increase its beds capacity, and most were able to transform their business models to corporations with profit motives and the ability to sell the business if it is not financially viable. It is not uncommon for conflicts to exist between a company's insatiable need for financial gain and the requirement to fulfill its corporate social responsibility—running a business for the common good.

Unlike other industries, the nursing home industry is unique in which the understanding of the concepts of "company profit motives" and "corporate social responsibility" are more applicable with regards to ethical and fair business practice. In nursing homes, there is a relationship that can be found, for example, in shortage of staff, resources, and financial investment impacting nursing home quality. Despite government oversight in operational/clinical issues, nursing homes are entrepreneurially self-directed on their reinvestment decisions. Hence, as long as there still exists incongruence between the huge government expenditure and the lack of return on investment in nursing home quality, one question will remain. Should the concept of corporate social responsibility be mandated in nursing homes?

Research shows that in fiscal year 2018, Medicaid expenditure was $407.6 billion, amounting to 3.5 percent of the national domestic product, with $1.1 trillion build-up expected in 2027. In an article titled "Nursing Homes as Complex Adaptive Systems: Relationship between Management Practice and Resident Outcomes," Anderson et al. (2007) observed that "despite numerous clinical and regulatory efforts, problems of poor quality of care in nursing homes continue, suggesting a need for effective management practices" (Wikipedia 2019, para 1).

Corporate entrepreneurs in nursing homes are expected to be self-conscious and self-directed to reinvest a fair amount of the resources to meet residents' and staff needs. And yet, like in anything else in life, bad entrepreneurial behavior such as greed is expected to rise for those who prefer higher profit margins in lieu of the necessary ploughing-back mechanisms. It is in this regard that Gordon and Stryker (1983, 71) wrote:

The administrator of a long-term care facility today is in an excellent position to creatively reintroduce into the lives of elderly residents opportunities for growth and personal enrichment. This cannot be done by role playing. Progress can and has been made by grasping and utilizing what history has taught, by leaving behind the dusty journals of institutional management which placed the welfare of the facility above the welfare of the residents.

Holistic nursing home management is concerned with the concept of proportionality, seeking a balance between subparts in the organizational systems. Increase in the corporate business models and the corporate chain formulations in the nursing home industry is likely to raise some eyebrows based on the inverse relationship still existing relative to nursing home quality, resident admissions equity, and government expenditures supporting nursing home operations.

In an article titled "The Changing Structure of the Nursing Home Industry and the Impact of Ownership on Quality, Cost, and Access," Hawes and Philips (1986, 19–36) described the trending "Corporatization," denoting its implication on the America healthcare system for acute care hospitals and long-term care facilities. The key observable points regarding long-term care facilities included the rapid increase in the cost of operating nursing homes compared to the acute care hospitals, and the rapid increase in the multi-facility chains since the 1970s.

For the holistic nursing home manager, there are two other issues worthy of note implicated in resident admissions equity. A discriminatory practice can occur in favor of admitting private-pay residents against admitting eligible Medicaid residents within the context of profit motives. Private-pay admissions tend to pay more than Medicaid. With specific reference to nursing home quality and admissions equity, it is stated that:

Critics of proprietary ownership generally speculate on the potential negative effects associated with the goal of profit maximization. They argue that a conflict may exist between the primary purpose of a proprietary business to show profit and the provision of high-quality care. Private-pay patients are more lucrative for nursing home owners because of Medicare and Medicaid payment limits (Hawes and Philips, 1986).

As the review of the corporate takeover of nursing homes continues, it is also noteworthy to cite some of its perceived advantages such as the ability to raise the initial business start-up private funds or funds to improve the business. The advantages and disadvantages associated with the ease by which private nursing home ownership can change hands remains debatable, but there seems to be no doubt of the psychosocial impact it has on residents and staff created by added uncertainties and new expectations. In most instances, when ownership changes hands, the incumbent facility administrators, staff, and residents are informed after the fact. Overall, it seems that there are still more questions than answers on the expectations that corporatization of nursing homes would bring private funds and management skills into the nursing homes to enable nursing home quality to increase, not decrease, and government funding to decrease, not increase

NHAs are frequently in a high-stakes decision-making role. They are licensed by their state governments to intervene and ensure fair play in financial management and regulatory compliance. Accordingly, each licensed nursing administrator is presented with a code of ethics issued by the Board of Examiners of Nursing Home Administrators of each state in the United States. The purpose of the code of ethics is to ensure that administrators manage their facilities in accordance with the state and federal governments' mandates, for which they are regulatory held accountable.

They have a wide range of responsibilities that affect every facet of the nursing home environment, as well as organizational commitment. The demands of a nursing home administrator require a leadership adeptness in all areas of operations of the facility, as well as highly capable team members who allow the NHA to act at the strategic management level. In an article titled "The Pivotal Role of the Nursing Home Administrator,"

Smikle (2014) posited that "moving beyond the academic, there is an important element of practicality in the discussion of the role the NHA plays in the facility and in the larger organization . . . sets the tone, establishes important aspects of organizational culture and models what is most important in terms of behavior and priorities" (Wikipedia 2019, para 2).

With reference to the function of the NHA, Sfantou et al. (2017), in an article titled "Importance of Leadership Style Towards Quality of Care Measures in Healthcare Settings: A Systematic Review," stated that "effective leadership of a healthcare professional is critical for strengthening quality and integration of care" (Wikipedia 2019, para 5). The concept of organizational integration through the nursing home administrator's leadership is recognized as crucial to improving and maintaining the nursing home quality within the facility. It involves the relationship between the administrator and every staff in the facility, as well as directing and coordinating the activities of the entire team to reach a mutual goal.

Quality of care is a critical factor in attaining high productivity levels within long-term care facilities. Sfantou et al. defined quality as "the degree to which the probability of achieving the expected health outcomes is increased and in line with updated professional knowledge and skills within health services."

There are eight styles of leadership that are more commonly seen in healthcare, and include transactional, translational, autocratic, laissez faire, task oriented, resonant, collaborative, and relationship oriented. Effective leadership is the key to achieving a high level of quality of care as well as successful patient outcomes (Sfantou et al).

An analysis of the effectiveness of the leadership styles showed that transformational and resonant leadership have resulted in reduced patient mortality, whereas relational and task-oriented leadership styles have been shown to significantly improve patient satisfaction (Sfantou et al). Also, transformational, transactional, and collaborative leadership resulted in improvement of patient satisfaction in both acute care and homecare. The goal of NHAs is to improve patient outcomes and reduce adverse incidents, which include unintentional injuries or complications that result in disability, death, and extended hospital stays, instead of the patient's primary condition.

Finally, leadership styles have been shown to illustrate the creation of organizational culture and the provision of effective patient care (Sfantou et al). Because of the necessity of holistic management in today's nursing homes and the importance of leadership as a change agent, more discussions about leadership are provided in the succeeding pages of this book

Utilizing Holistic Management within Functional Departments in Nursing Homes

A nursing home is comprised of a variety of functional departments that come together to provide quality and safe healthcare to the residents in the holistic perspective. These departments include the nursing units, pharmacy, medical records, social services, physical and occupational therapy, and management. All effort must be made to avoid strict departmental philosophy from obstructing the necessity for departmental cooperation and integrated efforts.

Combining holistic management practices with traditional ones into a companywide integration strategy and management can be a challenge (Johannsen, 2013). In order to integrate the two approaches in management, an integration scenario needs to be created and established (Johannsen). When developing a scenario, there is a specific motivation to choose integration strategies (Johannsen, 2013). There are various characteristics that a scenario can have:

- **Motivation:** New methods are combined with existing ones. There are synergies and weaknesses between the methods that are reduced by integration, and one is the prerequisite for the other.
- **Objects:** Integration of methods, including TQM, Six Sigma, LSCM, and AI.
- **Situation:** Project-related or project-independent integration.
- **Form:** Merging or joining.

Johannsen (2013, 1004) created a scenario to illustrate the integration of LSCM and Six Sigma quality management methods while striving for synergies between methods. The following is their description of their scenario:

> *Quality techniques are part of quality management methods, so that solely focusing on techniques would restrict the range of application for the integration approach too much. The quality management methods are to be integrated independent from a specific project constellation. By that it can be guaranteed, that the integrated method can be used for different improvement projects, while it can be adapted for different contexts after the integration has been performed. The methods are to be merged, which means that the integration results in one integrated method. The problems in coordinating different quality management methods have been described in literature. In addition, employees appreciate using one method for quality management while no problem of selecting a method is given. The integration approach to be developed focuses the integration of two methods at a particular time, which reduces complexity.*

Nursing home managers need to search for ways to integrate the strengths of holistic and traditional approaches. Like the quarterback in the American football team, one of the skills a holistic nursing home administrator needs to have is being able to visualize the whole field of play and to cultivate teamwork among his players necessary to win. It is easy to find arguments about which functional department is more important than the other. Such argument and self-aggrandizement is not in keeping with the tradition of holistic nursing home management or resident-centered care. The holistic nursing home management and resident-centered care is concerned with the importance of the resident's total well-being in accordance with the resident assessment and plan of care. A functional department is only important if its contribution to the individual resident has been identified in the resident care plan. What this concept means is that while one functional department may be hugely important in one setting, it may be minimally important in another. Therefore, it is important to revisit the departmental branding that existed in the traditional nursing home management to determine its efficacy under the holistic nursing home management.

Every healthcare organization is facing cuts in insurance reimbursements and penalties for certain adverse effects or complications. Some of the ways that a holistic management strategy can improve the organizational function in nursing home care quality outcomes include analyzing data on the organization's spending, determining the effects of health care reform on the financial status, involving all professional staff in planning meetings, and including stakeholders as much as practicable in decisions.

When utilizing holistic methods, administrators need to see the whole picture of the facility, not just one aspect, but how each part relates to one another. Optimizing cost savings is important to every administrator to keep the facility running, but there are other issues equally important, such as staffing, clinical and support services equipment, that must be considered. Reducing shifts or hours for nurses, aides, and other support services can be cost saving that increases profit margin, but patient care as it relates to nurse/patient ratios must remain a priority. Integration of holistic management into traditional standards of care takes a commitment of the entire organization, as well as a detailed plan regarding its implementation.

According to the Centers for Disease Control (CDC) article titled "Nursing Homes and Assisted Living (Long-term Care Facilities [LTCFs])," there are approximately 4 million people residing in nursing homes and skilled nursing facilities each year in the US, and about "1 to 3 million serious infections occur every year in these facilities" (Wikipedia 2018, para 1).

NHAs, who are strategically minded regarding cost, need to consider the entire picture when making cost-savings changes in the facility. An example of this is when comparing the cost of safety syringes to a non-safety one. It may cost more; however, if the rate of needle sticks are reduced, it's worth spending the extra amount rather than having to treat an employee for hepatitis B or C or HIV. Improvement of the patients' experiences or outcomes, as well as the financial status of the facility, is the targeted goal of most nursing homes.

NHAs have differing roles when comparing types of organizations, and they have critical ramifications for the ways an NHA has to prepare in order to successfully fulfill a management position. Those who work in management positions where they have little to no involvement in the finances of the organization need to have different skills than those who oversee every financial area of the nursing home. When changing management approaches in a nursing home, they cannot be done in a vacuum; every employee, from nurses to CEOs and social workers to pharmacists, need to be a part of the change, whether they are financial or procedural.

Because of the growing concerns about nursing home quality, administrators, in conjunction with their governing boards, will have to rethink their approaches to managing their facilities. Cost containment or the requirement to "do more with less" is a huge issue, as are patient outcomes. And those managers who are able to improve both through the integration of holistic principles with the traditional industry standards will be more successful in creating an environment that is both positive for the residents and minimizes adverse events. The ultimate goal of every facility is to provide quality care and safe conditions for all patients, as well as maintaining a financial plan that effectively meets the needs of the organization.

A nursing home administrator is oftentimes described as the person in charge of the daily operation of the nursing home. He is licensed by the state board of nursing home administrators, which can revoke his license for cause, but it is the governing body of the nursing home that hires and can fire the nursing home administrator. Accordingly, there exists a dual mandate in accountability process that is sometimes precarious for most administrators regarding their struggle to avoid conflicts of interest in their decision-making.

Regardless of the legal status of the nursing home (for profit, not for profit, or private), group decision-making between the governing body, the administrator, and other clinical staff is more likely to produce a favorable outcome if participation and discussions were open and factual. One of such sticky situations requiring group decision is the budgetary decision, the profit margin and its effect on nursing home quality.

The traditional organizational chart clearly shows the administrator as technically reporting to the governing board, but in practice, he is regarded as the middleman between the regulatory agencies or the state board, the governing body, and the direct care givers. He is in charge of coordinating and integrating activities relating to regulatory, legal, and financial compliance needed to avoid conflict of interest and achieve success in the holistic management perspective. The administrator must recognize that despite the top-down organizational management designed by Daniel McCallum (1815–1878), managing modern nursing homes has taken up new meaning and expectations, requiring administrators who are and would be more hybrid in their approach to management. According to most literature reviews, nursing home administration is defined as:

> *"A specialized area of medical and health services management. Nursing home administrators work to supervise nursing clinical and administrative affairs of nursing homes and related facilities . . . typical duties of nursing home administrators include overseeing staff and personnel, financial matters, medical care medical supplies, facilities, and other duties as specific positions demand" (Wikipedia, 2018, para 1).*

In general, nursing home administrators have extensive and demanding job descriptions, but to be a holistic administrator, he must understand how to be a leader as well as a manager of his organization. Leadership and management are two different concepts, even though we cannot do with one without the other. To be a holistic administrator implies the ability to apply leadership as well as managerial skills toward team building to manage change and motivate subordinates.

In an article titled "What Is Leadership?" Warren G. Bennis (1925–2014) provided the difference between being a leader and being a manager, and stated "leaders are people who do the right thing; managers are people who do things right." Dwight D. Eisenhower (1890–1969) shed more light on the definition of leadership with this quote: "leadership is the art of getting someone to do something you want done because he wants to do it" (Wikipedia, 2019, para 1–2). Deduced from both of these statements, as they apply to a holistic nursing home administrator, is the importance of vision and motivation-vision to see the future clearly and manage change and motivation to inspire others in the process of getting things done. We have already documented how much nursing homes have progressed from almshouses to its modern status through changes that came from regulatory and legislative means to assure improved administrative and clinical management in these institutions.

To continue to shape internal organizational relationships and structures in the holistic management perspectives, we need administrators who can develop new and specific administrative skills that assure effective answers to the demands of both the state boards and governing boards.

In real life, we hear the cliché involving the chicken and the egg, which came first? The administrator's relationship with the state board and the governing board demands that there is a clear understanding in upholding the federal, state, and municipal regulations as supreme by all parties, and the need for cooperative action by all to make things better. It is noteworthy that nursing home administrators understand that even though the holistic management model may not be enshrined as an organizational chart involving either of the boards, its form is behavioral based on staff attitudes and abilities to cultivate effective interpersonal relationships, teamwork, team morale, decision-making, and communication across the organizational spectrum. His ability manage change and to harmonize formal and informal organizational apparatus into one meaningful framework are important steps toward the achievement of holistic management.

Essentials of Decision-making and Holistic Management in Nursing Homes

Personal or organizational decision-making is an important part of our daily lives and the cornerstone in holistic management. Because the decisions we make have real-life consequences, they require careful deliberations that span the past, the present, and the future on the subject matter, devoid of interferences. Nursing home administrators are hired to make intuitive or rational decisions as an important part of their daily job function. It is important that his intuition and rationality in decision-making are not limited or controlled by external forces but by their management skills, knowledge of the industry, and human empathy.

In 1978, Herbert Simon theorized the concept of "bounded rationality" as applicable to decision-making and as a wake-up call to organizational decision makers, particularly those who are embarking in holistic management, to denounce any limitation that prevents our ability to make good decisions. Even though in bounded rationality Simon posited that "in decision making, rationality of individuals is limited by the information they have, the cognitive limitation of their minds, and the finite amount of time they have to make a decision" (Wikipedia, 2018, para 10), he never implied those conditions to be static. Simon's introduction of the concept of "satisficing" in 1956, therefore, pointed to human condition and circumstances when decision makers are forced to accept solutions that are less than optimum. He defined satisficing as "a decision making strategy or cognitive heuristic that entails searching through the available alternatives until an acceptability threshold is met," and stated, "decision makers can satisfice either by finding optimum solutions for a simplified world, or by finding satisfactory solutions for a more realistic world" (Wikipedia, 2018, para 1). Simon's theories are hoped to be a teaching moment in the pursuit of the new frontier in holistic nursing home management where quality of care outcomes are directly proportional to the quality of the decisions we make.

Oftentimes, when we analyze the differences in life's phenomena, most explanations always reflect an African proverb which states "all fingers are not the same." It is also true that when human beings are created, they are endowed by their creator with limitless potentials to expand the horizon of their thinking, abilities, skills, and knowledge on which their lot in life depends. Accordingly, when a decision maker adopts the cliché such as "I have done my best with what I have," he is accepting the defeatist attitude of choosing an easy way out, unwillingness to apply the extra effort needed to consider all possibilities in the process of optimizing his decision. The concept of "intractability" as a factor against good decisions can be man-made for those individuals who choose to become decision "satisficers" rather than decision "maximizers" in their decision-making process.

In an article titled "Satisficing vs Maximizing," Heshmat (2015) assessed the advantages and disadvantages of both concepts in decision-making and wrote, "when we face too many attractive choices, we can feel anxious about missing out. Satisficers are individuals who are pleased to settle for a good enough option, not necessarily the very best outcome. Overall, maximizers achieve better outcome than satisficers" (Wikipedia 2020, para 1–7).

While the premise of bounded rationality as propounded by Herbert A. Simon in 1947 can be regarded as substantive in behavioral science, decision makers do not have to subject themselves totally to its supposition. Maximizing an organizational or a personal decision is a challenging undertaking demanding adequate time, attention to details, sufficient research on the subject matter, information gathering, innovation, and mental alertness.

There are helpful hints in overcoming bounded rationality to make good organizational decisions. In an article titled "Three Approaches to Deal with Bounded Rationality," Doddi, (2018, 2) reflected on Shunryu Suzuki's concept of zen mind, beginner's mind, or the "beginner's mindset," essentially referring "to having an open mind without preconceptions when learning something even if you are an expert. If we are bounded in our rationality, then beginner's mind helps us to become boundless. In the beginner's mind there are many possibilities; in the expert's mind there are few."

Group decision-making has also been found to have a corrective effect on bounded rationality regarding information and cognitive and time deficits known to impede the assurance of making an optimizing decision. The two advantages in group over individual decision-making are synergy and information sharing, in which the collective effort ultimately produces a more effective decision. Groups that are cohesive, cooperative, and integrative do not only borrow from one another, they supplement one another to achieve not only their common goal but also individual self-fulfillment.

In every supportive group, the "good neighbors" concept of "what you do not have you can borrow from me" is aptly applicable. Organizational or personal decision-making within the good-neighbors concept has a value-added effect on decision outcomes in that "two heads are better than one" regarding information sharing that produces a wider knowledge base on the subject matter. Insufficient information on the issue for which a decision is required has already been cited as a limitation to the efficacy of the decision outcomes.

In 1989, a study that was conducted to determine whether or not the decisions made by Nigerian secondary school seniors to pursue or not to pursue higher education met their career needs and manpower development needs is an example. This study found students' decisions to be faulty and not in compliance with their personal or national socioeconomic development needs. Students were found to be uninformed of their felt needs and that of their society so that for the most part, "more students aspired to jobs than intended to major in those areas or vice versa" (Umoren, 1989).

It is philosophically arguable that it is through the process of decision-making that human beings find meaning that lies between human wisdom, knowledge, and benefits of good decisions. Adopting holistic management that is a decision-based management approach is not only an inspirational innovation in contemporary nursing homes, it is a regulatory mandate in the United States for participation in the Medicare and Medicaid program that "each resident must receive and the facility must provide . . ." (OBRA '87). This mandate is implicated in a web of critical and organized decision-making processes to achieve nursing home quality. Nursing home decisions are noted to be qualitative, quantitative, as well as comprehensive, for which the well-being of the residents and staff is affected.

The importance of defining a clear objective, alternative courses of action, and the expected outcome of these decisions has been discussed. Accordingly, there are two critical domains of nursing decisions. First, we have the domain of clinical decisions of direct care givers that have direct impact on resident care, and second, we have management decisions made by the governing board that have indirect impact on the entire nursing home as a business enterprise.

OBRA '87 mandates that each nursing home must have a governing board with accountability that the nursing home is legally, ethically, and morally constituted; and that its decisions relating to resource management, policy formulation, budgets, resident care and resident environmental standards, staffing, and oversight are in concert with the mission of its business type.

In either case, it is the responsibility of the licensed nursing home administrator to ensure balance to avoid substandard operation in the nursing home. For example, in today's nursing homes it is critical that there is an administrative decision that advocates for sufficient trained staff and sufficient medical, nursing, and environmental supplies if the holistic resident-centered care is to be achieved. Staffing and supply costs being noted as determining factors between profit and loss margins, high standard or substandard care, they have also been found as the root cause for poor care and consumer complaints. This realization has prompted state agencies to set minimum staffing standard for direct care givers (licensed nurses and certified nursing assistants) for which quantitative data is collected as part of the nursing home star-rating process throughout the United States.

The qualitative collection and analysis of data of nursing home staffing is still elusive. Nursing home regulations, however, mandate that nursing aides be given performance evaluations yearly. The assumption is that management understands the link existing between staff work performance rating and nursing home quality, and would be consistent in staff supervision and evaluation as a means of reeducating staff or removing them from the workforce for not providing quality care to residents.

Essentials of Communication and Holistic Management in Nursing Homes

Akin to the importance of decision-making, is the importance of an effective communication in propelling holistic nursing home management to achieve its goal of integrating stakeholders. As it was previously indicated, shared information, views, and ideas to achieve organizational goal, helpful in organizational decision-making, constitute the definition of organizational communication. In a book titled *Interpersonal Communication in the Modern Organization*, Bormann et al. (1969,

1) stated that "all organizations are held together by, and perform their functions through, interpersonal communication." McCroskey (2005), in an article titled "The Nature of Communication in Organization," stated "regardless of the type of organization, communication is the element that maintains and sustains relationships in it" (Wikipedia 2020, para.1).

Even though most social scientists have shown the essential types of organizational communication to include formal, informal, downward, upward, horizontal, oral, verbal, or written, organizations always have options to adopt the best fit for their unique situation. Nevertheless, because of the uniqueness of the nursing home operation and the tenet of holistic management, more of upward and horizontal communications, known for teambuilding, are encouraged, with sufficient attention to be paid to the informal communication or grapevine. If what employees and stakeholders are saying in private is not addressed in public, it can have a long-run effect on the organization as a whole.

The traditional formal top-down communication channels—usually existing in the form of meetings, conferences, telephone calls, company newsletters, and performance reviews—has its place in periodically connecting members of large-scale organizations. In whatever type of communication is consciously chosen, it should be noted that in nursing homes the reality is that there are more people at the bottom of this organizational pyramid whose work have direct impact on the population that they serve, requiring that their input and consultation be worthy of consideration in decision-making.

Millett (1966, 115–116), in his book titled *Organization for the Public Service*, wrote:

> *Communication is not a one-way street. Many administrators are likely to think of communication as the issuance of orders, directives, and instructions. Communication is also a matter of obtaining information, and analyzing its importance or significance correctly. We are often told that in a hierarchical organizational communication from top to bottom, or from the center outward to the*

fringes of the enterprise, tends to be critical; while communication from below toward the center tends to be complimentary . . . all groups or persons in an organization want to feel that their ideas are given some consideration. They want to know also that their experience in doing the work assigned to them is understood by their supervisors, and has been taken into account in the decisions which are made. Frequent contact between work groups and management is important in creating this sense of participation.

Millett expressed his preference for a two-way street communication, and encouraged that those individuals or groups in the communication channel should participate in the decision-making process.

Progressing from the traditional model of managing nursing homes to the holistic management model requires a change in the communication model in which information, views, and ideas are shared with stakeholders inside and outside the nursing home. Effective communication is important during organizational change to inform and educate stakeholders, and to encourage their commitment, participation, buy-in, and feedback.

In an article titled "Effective Communication Brings Successful Organizational Change," Husain (2013) wrote about stages and objectives of communication during change in organization as consisting of the "unfreezing stage, move stage" and the "refreezing stage . . . build structures and processes that support the new ways" (Wikipedia 2018, para 44). Each of the stages is designed separately to prepare staff and other stakeholders in the implementation and management of change and communication of uncertainties in caregiving.

A nursing home is a people- and service-oriented organization in which most of its interested clientele also located outside the nursing home stands to benefit from effective planning for change. Holistic nursing home management thrives on establishing effective communication channels and information flows between residents, employees, families, and the community. Holistic nursing home management requires an expansion in scope and frequency of communication with stakeholders. A free flow of information, views, and ideas on change and during caregiving is more likely to create a more inclusive, educated, and enlightened system, and nursing home quality can be examined within a proper context without the blame game stemming from misunderstanding.

The holistic nursing home management approach emphasizes three types of interrelated communication modules that exist in nursing homes, which are noteworthy to all administrators. The leadership communication is designed to communicate organizational policies and instructions to staff; inter-staff communication is designed to share information about caregiving and their needs; and staff-to-resident communication is designed to create staff/resident relationships and bonding.

In an article titled "How Effective Communication with Long-Term Care Staff Achieves the Best Care," Terrace (2015) wrote: "establishing effective communication between LTC staff, residents and their families helps to provide the type of care that is most responsive to residents' needs, values and preferences . . ." (Wikipedia, 2020, para 2). Significantly, staff communication encounters with the residents must emphasize respect, empathy, and dignity that create not only a partnership between staff and residents, but a foundation for excellent resident care.

Chapter 7

Integrating LTC Regulations with Facility Policies, Programs, Processes, and Practices as a Function of Holistic Management in Nursing Homes

The importance of nursing home policy covering "resident care and personnel" cannot be overemphasized. Government regulations and its strict oversight in nursing homes began when OBRA '87 set forth its minimum standard of care. Consequently, nursing homes would need facility policies and procedures to help them fulfill the government mandate stating that "the facility will be administered in a manner that enables it to use its resources effectively and efficiently to attain and maintain the highest practicable physical, mental and psychological wellbeing of each resident."

There is a special relationship existing between LTC government regulations and a facility's policies, programs, process, and practices that can't be overlooked. All nursing home policies, programs, processes, and practices are purported to be derived in a synchronizing fashion from the LTC government regulations and community practices. In recent years, the earlier belief that regulating nursing homes alone could be the be-all and end-all in delivering nursing home quality has been questioned. Government LTC regulations are directives and guidelines requiring that they are effectively implemented by nursing homes practitioners. Harkins (2014) in an article titled "The Broken Promise of OBRA '87: The Failure to Validate the Survey Protocol," citing the inefficiency in the inspection process, to name a few, wrote "Nursing facilities are among the most heavily regulated entities in the American economy. Unfortunately, nursing facilities also are among the most inconsistently and ineffectively regulated entities . . . government inspections of facilities do not result in valid, accurate, and consistent assessments of the quality of care" (Wikipedia 2020, para 1).

How nursing homes became heavily regulated cannot be viewed in a vacuum. Research findings on nursing home quality as posited in many parts of this book has confirmed that complaints and rumors of resident abuse and neglect in nursing homes had become rampant, causing lawmakers to act, or overreact, with more regulations. Consequently and in accordance with holistic management, there seems to exist many thought-provoking questions to be answered pertaining the nature and history of nursing homes as human organizations, the overall management approach in nursing homes, the effectiveness of nursing home government regulations and inspections, the right amount of government regulations, as well as the type of improvement in government regulations needed to improve nursing home quality.

While it is true that government regulations are well intentioned to improve nursing home quality, there are some misgivings that nursing homes may be overburdened by regulations, government oversight, and inspections. Nursing home government inspection is seen as an after-the-fact data collection activity while poor care affecting residents, causing pain and suffering, is either existent or ongoing and needs a proactive, not a reactive plan. It is our belief that the goal of these multitudes of direct resident care regulations in nursing homes is to "comprehensively" help improve the care residents receive.

It is also apparent that at this juncture nursing homes may benefit from nursing home intra-organizational reform. When we look at nursing home management strictly from a medical-disease model, we have missed a chunk from the promise of holistic nursing home management. The basic assumption that needs to be understood by all stakeholders in nursing homes is that whatever medical condition a resident may have is constant, but it is the behavior of human beings that would make the problem better or worse.

The second question to ask pertains to how much nursing home operators are viewing the facility's policies, programs, processes, practices, staff training, and staff supervision as they affect resident care outcomes and facility compliance. The third question to ask pertains to the administrator's leadership alongside the governing board in developing and implementing meaningful resident care policies and staff handbook that are derived from the holistic management perspective and LTC regulations for each nursing home. It is therefore not recommended that corporations with multiple nursing homes use generic policies or policies not developed to target the configurations and needs of each nursing home, its residents and staff. Also, it would be wrong, though not uncommon, for employees who work in different nursing facilities to borrow and use policies that are not designed for that particular facility. Developing effective and meaningful facility policies and procedures that reflect holistic management, targeting LTC regulations and synchronizing them with programs, processes, and practices, can be considered as an important part of management functions requiring practice, expertise, and administrative dexterity. Therefore, the use of an LTC expert to lead the group is advisable to avoid the "blind leading the blind," since a facility policies and procedures are often considered not only the organizational unifying force but also what gives a collective and individual direction within the organization.

In emulating holistic management approach, the best practice is that facility policies and procedures developed or revised cooperatively among organizational members and their leadership are much easier to implement and more apt to produce successful outcomes than those off-the-rack policies. The holistic management principles technically require the input of employees in all aspects of managing human organizations to include the organizational culture of the facility. The presumption is that staff who do the work and had participated in developing their organizational policies and procedures are more likely not only to remember the policies and procedures that they wrote but also would be more motivated to use them in the intended areas of care.

The fact remains that during the process of developing a particular policy, staff would have had the opportunity to ask the why, how, what, when, and where questions needed in the development of effective nursing home policies and procedures. The benefit of creating a sense of ownership and inclusiveness among organizational stakeholders is the ability of management to legitimize the effort and elicit employees' participation and collaboration to achieve organizational goals.

The fundamentals of adult learning are based on group participation and task orientation, where the group decides for themselves what will work or will not work in guiding their path to their project success. With this understanding, the holistic nursing home administrator would have succeeded in building a team around something of interest to the team, something enjoyable to do or use; something that is more practical and easier to memorize to avoid the inconvenience of the frequent attempts to refer to the "cheat sheet" or use shortcuts in the facility's policy and procedures to address certain concerns.

Staff should be encouraged to "follow and apply" facility policies in their entity and as was written for that particular facility. Not following facility policies and procedures the way it was determined has serious consequences. While government regulations for nursing homes are designed to set minimum standards, a facility's policies are written to establish the road map on how to consistently achieve those standards. When that happens, the facility has a better chance of meeting regulatory standards consisting of federal, state, and local. For example, for nursing home physicians under "physician supervision," it is required that the admitting physician certifies all residents admitted into the nursing home in writing, and they will continue to supervise their care for their entire duration of stay. But it is through an administrative decision of the nursing home per its policy that requires certain time frames for which each activity must be completed, understanding that the facility can be held regulatorily and legally accountable if the time frames it sets are not upheld or are inconsistent with the community norms.

Secondly, as a general rule, if your facility policy says you should proceed with your activity using A, B, and C, in that order, it would be a command, not an option. But if an employee chooses to proceed with B to C without A and an adverse effect results, the employee and his facility can be held liable. Nursing home administrators who embrace holistic management must also ensure that all operational policies and procedures in their facilities are reviewed and revised periodically to reflect holistic management principles in supervisory management, as well as changes in government regulations.

Developing and mastering facility policies and procedures are important adjuncts to behavior management in a human organization, which guides the delivering of quality care through experiential learning. The proponents of experiential learning, also called hands-on learning, include John Dewey, Kurt Lewin, and Jean Piaget. Aristotle (384–322 BC) wrote, "for the things we have to learn before we can do, we learn by doing them." Not having organizational policies and procedures to guide or regulate the behavior of organizational members can be compared to driving a car on a road where there are no stop signs, no lane separations, no traffic lights, no speed limits, and expecting not to have an accident. "Workplace policies establish boundaries, guidelines and best practices for acceptable behavior at your business. The purpose of policies such as these is they allow you to communicate to your employees the way you expect them to behave on the job" (Wikipedia 2019, para 3). It is also noted that "a policy is a deliberate system to guide the decision and achieve rational outcomes" (Wikipedia 2019, para.1).

Beyond being a guide to quality care, policies can also be useful tools for lawyers and families when filing grievances against the nursing home. Ellerman (2016), in an article titled "Why Nursing Home Policies and Procedures Are So Important," wrote,

> *when families call our office about an incident that occurred in a Virginia nursing home, one that appears to the family as neglect, or worse, abuse, we often encourage the family to request a copy of the facility policies related to the incident. For an example, the fall policies. The assessment policies. The nutrition policies. Change in condition policies. That way we can investigate the case, and frankly the allegations of negligence with the written policies as a backdrop. Truthfully, they can be a tremendously helpful map for patients' families during care, and during litigation (Wikipedia 2019, para 6).*

Because of what policies in and of themselves mean to every organization, nursing homes included, the quality of every policy should be strictly considered during its development. A well-developed policy must be organization or industry specific, goal specific, easy to read, easy to follow in a step-by-step process, assessable to end users, and reflecting the targeted regulation or law that the organization is intending to uphold. In the main, facility policies in nursing homes are formulated to cover four main areas relating to resident quality of care, quality of life, resident environment per regulations, and "employee conduct" labor laws. In an article titled "30 Essential Policies and Procedures for Long-term Care," subtitled "Relationship to Other Department of Health and Human Services Regulations," Burke (2006) posited that facilities are required to "implement policies and procedures in order to address its obligations to meet the applicable provisions of other HHS regulations" (Wikipedia, 2019, para 1). The other provisions referred herein relate to facilities having policies to forbid or prevent discrimination based on race, color, national origin, handicap, age, human subject of research, fraud, and abuse, notably in employment, housing, and health.

Having a comprehensive knowledge of the sources of nursing home regulations in developing facility resident-related policies and the employee handbook is critical for a holistic nursing home administrator, alongside understanding the linearity that exists between source documents in law, the legislative process, the details of nursing home regulations, the art of developing nursing home policies and management practices, to ensure compliance with legal and regulatory requirements. The concept of linearity in general emphasizes how one thing relates to another, with traceability to its origin. Therefore, to the nursing home administrators whose job function is explaining regulations, enforcing regulations, developing nursing home policies and practices, understanding the concept of linearity in health law is noteworthy and helpful when it comes to applying each law or regulation fairly and effectively.

It must be noted that the job description of a holistic nursing home administrator is the assumption that they are aware of their authority, responsibility, and accountability relative to their supervisory role over residents and staff. Therefore, for all residents who live in nursing homes and employees who work there, there must be a written document that entitles them, under the law, to the basic protection against abuse and neglect. For example, the civil rights laws and policies representing the source of freedom for all citizens in every facet of American society, including those residing in nursing homes, is traceable to or derived from the Constitution and the Bill of Rights. Similarly, in nature, the offspring of the same species owes its existence and meaning to its ancestry in keeping with the axiom that the fruit does not fall far from its tree. This argument is applicable to societies where the rule of law is linked to the Constitution or the common law as the foundation for an effective governance, human rights, and management practice.

When human beings find connectivity in their daily activities of life, they will simultaneously find order and reason to perceive life in general as meaningful. It is within this context that the constitutional law or the common law exists, which:

> *Defines the role, powers, and structure of different entities within a state, namely, the executive, the parliament or legislative, and the judiciary; as well as the basic rights of citizens and, in federal countries such as the United States and Canada, the relationship between the central government and state, provincial, or territorial government (Wikipedia, 2019 para.1).*

Under our system of a democratic government and jurisprudence, laws are designed to regulate different sectors of our socioeconomic life, health, and welfare, and to protect all citizens regardless of their gender, religion, race, or national origin. Many branches of the law that protect citizens and regulate our socioeconomic behaviors are criminal laws, labor laws, civil rights laws, contract and healthcare laws, to name a few. Some of these laws exist in the form of written documents such as the United States Constitution, and others exist in the form of unwritten common laws based on tradition, such as in the United Kingdom. Notable is the extent to which healthcare laws in the United States and elsewhere borrow from the different aspects of the total body of laws that exist in that society, oftentimes traceable to the constitutional acts of Congress or common law.

To a holistic nursing home practitioner, it is necessary to understand the origin of healthcare laws and how the different aspects of laws coexist to provide the total protection of nursing home residents and staff as citizens. Whenever a wrongful act is committed in nursing homes involving resident or staff and a lawsuit is filed, it is most likely that not only is their contract with the institution violated, but other laws also traceable to either the constitution or common law itself. In other words, health care laws cannot be viewed in isolation. They cannot be incongruent with either the constitution or the common law. The intent of the legislation cannot be misunderstood, nor can they be subjected to misinterpretation or contradiction in relation with state or county laws. Healthcare regulations exist in agreement with the constitution or common law, not in spite of it.

It is within this basic understanding that Litka and Inman (1975, 119) posited that:

> *Law prescribes the environment in which society functions and it suggests guidelines for individuals to carry on their daily activities. Law similarly defines the rights and liberties of individuals within society, and the rights of society in regards to its members. In its present form, law is the result of many years of change and a concerted effort to keep social controversy within limits. Under any scheme of social order, the first concern of society should be for the security of the individual. And, because of the many races and many creeds that make up our society, it was felt necessary to shield many types of life, character, opinions and beliefs . . . Where conduct of any party is wrongful to another, the aggrieved party is entitled to seek legal relief. Where wrongful conduct interferes with the interests of society In general, it may be classified as criminal and subjected to sanctions that society might impose.*

In the United States, the Constitution, which was written in 1776, is the supreme law of the land. It gives powers to different branches of government—the executive, the legislature, and the judiciary—within the federal, state, and local governments. Its tripartite or tri-federal nature also grants the states, counties, and municipalities the rights and freedoms to enact their own laws, including healthcare laws, based on self-determination and culture.

The Tenth Amendment to the US Constitution explains "Federal laws are generally applicable in the same way across all state borders . . . This is because every U.S. state is also a sovereign entity in its own right and is granted the power to create laws and regulate them according to their needs." Even though healthcare laws are not directly specified as a civil right in the US Constitution, it is implied within the Bill of Rights, enabling each state or local legislature to enact and implement all laws, including healthcare laws, as long as they do not conflict with the federal ones. LTC surveyors are trained to traverse these demarcation lines between federal, state, and county laws to provide proper surveillance, inspections, findings, interpretation, and penalties based on applicable laws.

It should be noted that while federal, state, and county/municipal laws have a common goal in mind to protect each resident's care needs, each law may be more stringent and definitive than the other. For example, treating residents with dignity during dining may imply the use of appropriate silverware. In an emergency, the use of paper plates are allowed unanimously even though some states may exclude the use of certain types of paper plates. It is important that a holistic nursing home administrator pay attention to the details between the federal, state, and county laws in developing and implementing their clinical, environmental policies and the employee handbook. Your employee handbook is important in defining the facility's workplace operating policies and procedures, and employees' expected personal conduct that all new employees must know and maintain for the duration of their employment. Lack of clarity and enforcement of these policies and procedures have been cited by many human resources writers as one of the sources of a toxic workplace. Most importantly, it is within the employee handbook that the rights of employers and employees are safeguarded. In our opinion, and given the nature and mission of nursing homes, an effective management of the workforce to avoid workplace toxicity should be one of the highest priorities of the holistic nursing home administrator.

Historically, governmental involvement in the American healthcare system dates back to the late 1600s due to its concerns for public health and safety as a matter of combating or controlling outbreaks of diseases and infections. Notably, it was the congressional act of 1798 that established the Marine Hospital Service to help disabled and sick marines. In 1804, the Boston Marine Hospital was built in Charleston for this purpose.

Legislative laws affecting healthcare or any aspect of the socioeconomic structure are derived directly or indirectly from the constitution, and crafted not to deviate from it. It is noteworthy that in most democracies like the United States, there are levels of government that are hierarchically connected, from federal to state and county, with different designations of law that embrace their jurisdictional uniqueness and diversity without conflicting with the constitution.

With respect to healthcare laws in general and nursing homes in particular, there are legislations reflecting the federal, state, county, and municipal standards. Through the Act of Congress, it is the Federal Department of Health and Human Service (HHS) that has the oversight on health, subcontracted to states to ensure compliance but allowing county and municipal governments to administer certain health laws pertaining to them. A holistic awareness of how healthcare laws are allocated and administered is required by the nursing home administrator to be able to keep the facility in compliance across federal, state, and municipal guidelines. Consequently, each state, county, and municipality is able to interpret, create, or apply its laws without violating the constitution or the federal statute.

The function of US Congress is to pass laws, either to start new programs or to improve the quality of the existing ones. The Social Security Act of 1935 and the Medicare and Medicaid Act of 1965 are examples of new initiatives that the US Congress passed into law to provide insurance protection for citizens against issues of poverty and/or health. The passage of the Medicare, Medicaid, and Social Security laws in the United States have been regarded as revolutionary, making it easy to manage national healthcare programs and other social service programs to provide relief to needy citizens. Research shows that over 64 million or one out of six Americans collected Social Security benefits in 2020, while in 2018, Medicaid provided health coverage to about 97 million low-income Americans and 10 million seniors with disabilities.

Chapter 8

The Matrix for Nursing Home Quality in the Holistic Management Perspective

According to the federal government mandate covering nursing homes in the United States, OBRA '87 and its basic requirement for Medicare/Medicaid participation (ROP), the prerequisite for nursing home quality (NHQ), is clearly documented. It demands that there is a thorough government oversight for an ethical operation of nursing homes, empowering care recipients to demand and receive continuous and empirical quality care that is multidimensional and comprehensive.

Consequently, and as previously mentioned, the matrix of nursing home quality has four (4) broad components consisting of resident quality of life (R-QOL), resident quality of care (R-QOC), resident quality of the environment (R-QOE), and resident fund management (RFM). Each component, having its own ingredients contributing to each resident's total well-being, has to be interrelatedly coordinated in keeping with the concept of resident-centered care and holistic management.

For clarity, and in almost all cases, R-QOL pertains to the social aspect of care, asking how much social activity, amenities, and freedom of choice are available for residents; R-QOC pertains to the clinical-medical aspect of care, asking how much clinical-medical attention the resident needs and receives; R-QOE pertains to the conduciveness of the physical plant and the human environment of care as it relates to resident safety and security, resident right for self-determination, respect, and dignity, to name a few; and RFM requires nursing homes to be ethical in resident fund management and to periodically provide accounting information to them.

The holistic nature of nursing management requires that all four areas of care for each resident be viewed as coequals in their contributions toward the resident's well-being. For example, the assumption that noncompliance in any aspect of these four areas of care is less traumatic to the resident means a major misunderstanding of OBRA's meaning of "comprehensive care."

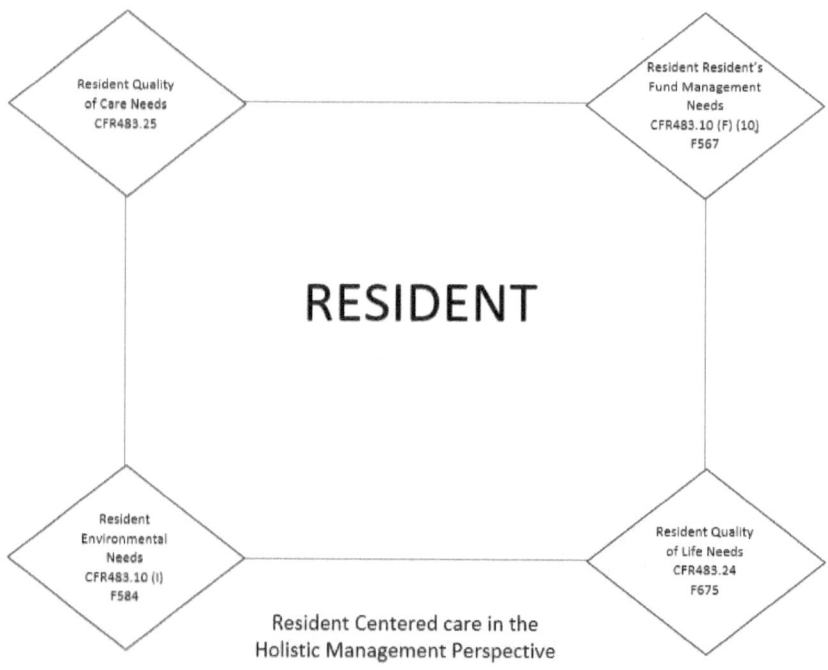

Resident Centered Care in the Holistic Management Perspective

Needs Structure	Some Related Components of Needs by Categories
SELF-ACTUALIZATION	Resident's rights · Meaning Creativity · Empowerment Competence · Spirituality Enrichment · Growth-Mentality Hope
ESTEEM NEEDS	Resident's rights · Self-Control Independence · Dignity, Privacy Empowerment · Identity Education · Coping/expression Self-respect · Self-respect Assertiveness · Decision making "Sexuality" (Sulloway, 1979, 283)
BELONGINGNESS/LOVE	Resident's rights · Family Contacts Community/organizational relationship Employee/resident relationship Resident/resident relationship Visitations Religious affiliation
SAFETY NEEDS	Resident's rights Physical/emotional security Property protection Financial protection Legal protection Medical attention for psychological and biological functioning Environmental safety Sanitation
PHYSIOLOGICAL NEEDS	Resident's rights · Food Water · Air Shelter · Exercise/activity Rest/comfort · Linen Personal Clothing

Components of Residents Care Needs along Maslow's Hierarchy of Needs Theory in nursing homes

Adapted from: Umoren (1992, 660) Maslow Hierarchy of Needs and OBRA 1987: Toward Needs Satisfaction by Nursing Home Residents Educational Gerontology: An International Journal, Volume 18, Number 6

Components of Residents Care Needs along Maslow's Hierarchy of Needs Theory in Nursing Homes

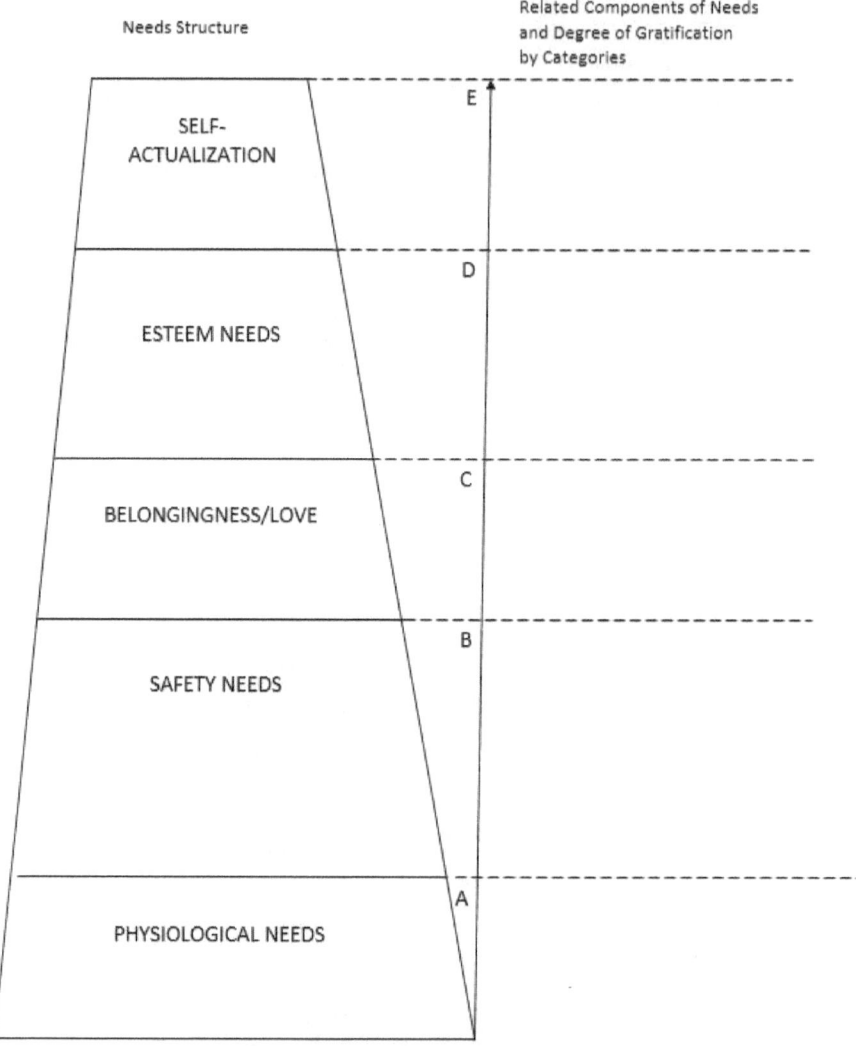

Needs Structure

Related Components of Needs
and Degree of Gratification
by Categories

E

D

C

B

A

SELF-
ACTUALIZATION

ESTEEM NEEDS

BELONGINGNESS/LOVE

SAFETY NEEDS

PHYSIOLOGICAL NEEDS

Degree of resident's need satisfaction along Maslow's Hierarchy of Needs
The core concept column on the right indicates where need gratification in A > B > C > D > E
(i.e., the smaller the area, the more the need therein is comparatively gratified.

Adapted from: Umoren (1992, 660) Maslow Hierarchy of Needs and
OBRA 1987: Toward Needs Satisfaction by Nursing Home Residents
Educational Gerontology: An International Journal, Volume 18, Number 6

Degree of Resident Needs Satisfaction Along
Maslow's Hierarchy of Needs Theory

Defining Resident Rights, Safety, Security, Dignity, Preference, and Self-determination in Holistic Nursing Home Management

In holistic nursing home management, optimizing each resident's total care is key. There is an interdependency of residents' needs satisfaction, caregivers' job performance, meeting residents' expectations, fulfilling employees' responsibility with accountability, and properly defining and treating residents with:

Respect and responsiveness
Encouragement and engagement
Service and supportiveness
Identity and intuitiveness
Dignity and devotion
Empathy and emotionality
Needs and nurture
Tenderness and transference
Sensitivity and sensibility

Accordingly, the term *resident quality of life* as contained in OBRA '87 implies assuring each resident's privacy, rights, safety, security, dignity, preferences, self-determination, to name a few, within the context of "comprehensive" care. In general, it is also accepted that the basic human needs in society include the need to feel safe and secure, to be treated with respect and dignity, to be able to make choices, decide on preferences, and to be able to search for life's meaning through self-determination. Nursing home residents are no exception. Pairing OBRA '87 with Maslow's hierarchy of needs theory and incorporating them into nursing home practice is intended to make residents' lives worthy and meaningful. In the main, resident safety in nursing homes is often discussed within the context of fire prevention, environmental hazard, resident falls, medication errors, resident abuse and neglect, developing pressure ulcers, loss of personal belongings, emotional distress coming from noise levels, and staff behavior affecting residents' health and well-being.

Safety and security mean two different things even though they have been used interchangeably, requiring a technical definition of each to ensure clarity of meaning and purpose. Some writers have described safety and security as two sides of the same coin. We view safety as the inner feelings that all human beings have regarding their protection from physical or emotional harm, while security is viewed as a shield or protocol that is in place and used to protect human beings from harm or danger. It should be noted that when nursing home residents feel unsafe, that feeling, rational or irrational, has the tendency to emotionally magnify due to residents' preexisting health conditions and their inability to self-help.

Being a holistic nursing home manager demands having a clear understanding of the implications of residents' safety and security, denoting that we cannot have one without the other. Taken together, they represent a holistic view of risk management designed to provide the security protocols that enhance the safety needs of residents. For example, on a rainy day we need the security of having the right size of umbrella to provide us safety from getting wet in the rain. Putting it another way, the presence of a meteorologist who gives the weather forecast represents the security we need in safety preparedness against inclement weather. It is essential that the holistic nursing home manager thoroughly understands the goodness of fit between security and safety, and the intensity in which they affect the well-being of citizens, especially those residing in nursing homes.

It should be noted that the amount of security- and safety-related protocols provided in nursing homes is directly proportional to the residents' felt need for safety but inversely proportional to residents' risk for physical and emotional harm. Alleviating the psychological fear among nursing home residents requires a holistic risk management program that encourages active and direct participation with families and all levels of staff.

Poor communications and decision-making about resident security and safety have serious implications. When adverse events are shared after the fact as a matter of "family notification," negative opinions and bad feelings about nursing homes multiply. On the other hand, when the holistic nursing home administrator is proactive with his risk management and safety information, sharing the residents' risk factors with families, residents, and staff, he is building a coalition of goodwill and trust among stakeholders.

The General Framework of Human Safety, Security, and Rights in Society

The need for humans to feel safe, secure, and that they have rights are a part of the social contract between citizens and society. Residents residing in nursing homes are citizens who are covered by the social contract. McCullough and Wilson (1995, 141) analyzed resident safety and security in nursing homes, calling it a value that is holistically related to other values and "ought to be understood within the context of other values." For the society at large, the belief in and the importance of safety and security remain the same. The absence of safety and security in society is related to general destruction and the concerns about potential physical or psychological harm or actual harm to humans, self-determination, lifestyle changes, duty to serve others, negligence, legal and non-legal remedies. In nursing homes, the investigation and interpretation of a resident's incident is not a matter of black and white but one that demands insightfulness and commitment to decide its cause and effect, even if the affected resident is in a state of incapacitation. Nevertheless, in nursing homes, safety issues that have caused or have the potential to cause harm to the resident or staff must be reported to an appropriate authority.

For humans, the need to feel safe and secure, with their rights and freedoms protected, is paramount in society and permeates all aspects of our lives. Feeling safe and secure in society is a felt need in everyone's life that cannot be purported to exist outside of our own perception and thoughts as interpreted by others. They can only be interpreted from within our own intrapersonal experience, expression, and values. For example, telling someone else that his own room temperature is adequate when he feels otherwise would be imposing, dictatorial, and not based on the principles of resident-centered care.

Human beings are endowed by their Creator with rights to life, liberty, and happiness, all implicated in safety and security for oneself. The US Constitution emphasized the protection of "life, liberty and property." When Plato (428–348 BC) theorized that a good life is possible only in a society, he echoed his sentiment of an ideal society, envisioning societies in which everyone lives in perfect harmony without fear of violence or worries about physical or emotional harm. The theory of an ideal society was followed thousands of years later by the theory of Utopianism. Thomas More's (1478–1535) description of utopia became the roundabout way of dismissing Plato's concept of an ideal society as fantasy and nonexistent. An ideal society is defined as an imaginary society where "the Giver is an example of a utopian society but at the same time reminds us that there is an obvious reason as to why our human nature will never allow it to work." Unlike the imaginary Utopia, which paints the picture of societies as the Garden of Eden, dystopia, on the other hand, describes societies of total anarchy where only pain and suffering exist.

In medieval times, it was commonplace to see societal phenomena in terms of either good or evil, heaven or hell. Today's societies are not exclusively good or bad, heaven or hell, but something in between; namely, managed societies. From the beginning of time and the expulsion of Adam and Eve from the Garden of Eden, the struggle with societal imperfections and the quest for its perfection in human safety and security have become rudimentary in holistic thinking in finding harmony and meaning within the context of the whole. We will begin with the understanding of safety and security as the cornerstone of well-being in all humans, including those who are institutionalized.

Accordingly, the holistic care for safety and security can be achieved when all citizens join hands in the struggle, from their own experience, to feel safe and secure, with rights to voice complaints if they otherwise feel unsafe, insecure, or fearful. Nursing home residents are citizens, and therefore are no exception. Safety and security are what they feel and express, requiring positive actions for change. Empowering them to determine their own aspirations and needs is the real of essence of life, encompassing the holistic care and caring for one and another.

As a general rule, human beings are guided by self -determination and personal preference to psychosocially exist under conditions that maximize the quality of their lives. As stated earlier, unfulfilled human needs for safety and security are detrimental to the fulfillment of other vital human needs, likely to provoke anxiety and depression in the elderly and among nursing home residents who may not be able to self-adjust.

Safety and security protection needs can be local, national, and international in scope, such as the spread of diseases and wars. COVID-19, which started in 2020, and WWII, which started in 1939, are clear examples of global jeopardy for safety and security. Historically, after WWII ended in 1945, the United Nations (UN) was formed to bring to an end the concerns for global safety and security, public or private. Because world wars were considered the number one threat to human safety and security, new global security alliances were formed. The United Nations (UN) was formed in 1945, which replaced the discredited League of Nations in 1946, and in 1949 NATO was formulated. The Warsaw Treaty Organization (WTO) and its Warsaw Pact (WP) were formulated in 1955. NATO comprised of global Western Bloc countries, while the Warsaw Pact comprised of global Eastern (former Soviet Union) Bloc countries, each acting as a check on the other to ensure global safety, security, and peace through balance of power.

The question is, what does global safety and security have to do with nursing home safety? The simple answer is that there is a trickle-down effect existing between global safety and national safety; anything that threatens the safety and security of the general population nationally is a double threat to nursing home residents who depend on others for their survival. Besides, in holistic management, the teaching is to look at the big picture and to seek connections existing in the organizational, national, or global phenomena. Accordingly, nursing homes in the United States are mandated, in addition to internal "fire and safety" plans, to have "external disaster plans," whose guidelines are contained in the CMS's ROP, requiring nursing homes to develop external disaster plans that are linked to the city and state Comprehensive Emergency Management Plan (CEMP).

In the United States, the concern for safety and security for all its citizens is deemed very important. The emergency 911 call was established in 1967, and the CEMP initiative, as adopted by OBRA, became law in 2016. These are a few examples of nationwide programs designed for human safety and security in the United States. On September 11, 2001, a watershed 911 event paralyzed the city of New York, putting every citizen at risk, including those residing in nursing homes, intensifying the mandate for all organizations to have an external emergency preparedness plan. Under nursing home guidelines, an external emergency preparedness plan must be reviewed or activated periodically to assure the state of readiness. Furthermore, the United Nations' thirty articles of the Universal

Declaration of Human Rights, published in 1948 as part and parcel of an international law, implied provisions for human safety and security. Accordingly, most global democracies have enshrined these articles in their constitutions to be followed by all organizations. In that sense, it is noteworthy that exercising human rights is implicated in safety guaranties, with legal provisions to support it. In nursing homes, information regarding resident safety, security, rights, and freedoms are outlined by CMS-related literatures and the ADA (Americans with Disabilities Act) of 1990. The ADA stipulates that "the facility must be designed, constructed, equipped, and maintained to protect the health and safety of residents, personnel and the public . . . the facility must meet the applicable provisions of the 2000 edition of the Life Safety Code of the National Fire Protection Association."

The NFPA (National Fire Protection Association) is the designated organization with safety and security guidelines to be followed to surveil physical environment in nursing homes. Nursing homes in the United States are inspected once a year at minimum by the local government authorities under the NFPA 101 Life Safety Code (LSC) as revised by CMS.

On resident rights, CMS stipulates that "resident has a right to a dignified existence, self- determination, and communication with access to persons and services inside and outside of the facility."

In holistic nursing home management, it is important to establish a link and meaning between security, safety, and rights. In other words, it is a violation of resident rights if the facility, through acts of omission or commission, fails to protect the resident from harm.

Requirement of Participation: Nursing Home Surveillance and Compliance in the Holistic Management of Nursing Homes

In general, nursing homes in the United States are inspected by state agencies to assure that the nursing home quality under the requirement of participation (ROP) in the Medicaid and Medicare programs is upheld to include safety and security precautions for the residents, visitors, and staff. While WWIII has thus far been prevented due to the implication of safety emphasized after WWII, concerns for public and individual safety, security, and human rights tend to be increasing, not decreasing.

Public and individual safety and security are not mutually exclusive. They both cause pain, suffering, physical disability, and even death to human beings without adequate safety and security precautions in place. Concern for public safety and security is a collective sense of fear from an expected or actual disaster that causes physical or emotional harm to masses of people. Some of the sources of public safety concerns relate to international conflicts; natural and industrial disasters; nuclear, chemical, and biological attacks; viruses; wildfires; infectious disease outbreaks; human trafficking; firearms attacks; and climate change.

In healthcare, particularly long-term care, concern for individual safety and security is an internalized sense of fear and vulnerability from expected or actual negative care outcomes. Areas of such concern are related to pain management, infections, medication errors, diagnosis, resident falls with injuries, pressure ulcers, delirium, dehydration, and poor environment management for residents with delirium, dementia, and frequent fallers due to other health reasons. Other areas of safety concern in nursing homes not frequently discussed are shortage of clinical staff, alarm hazards, health information technology (HIT), and workplace violence.

The impact of nurses shortages in nursing homes is concerning with regards to safety risks and as a barrier to holistic health management. Also, in some situations, some nursing home staff found to be desensitized by frequent nurse call bell or fire alarm rings do fail to respond, hence creating a safety risk for the residents. HIT is another area where safety risk can occur due to its newness in nursing homes. While there are as many proponents as opponents to HIT, it is yet clear how HIT in nursing homes supports the definition of staff productivity, especially for those residents who depend on human beings for turn and position, feeding, ambulation, and so forth. Limited staff training and distractions caused by heavy caseloads have been cited for poor or missed clinical documentation and health information being exposed to unauthorized persons. While the possibility for staff/staff or resident/resident or staff/resident altercations exists in a crowded dual-utility environment like the nursing home, the holistic manager must work to prevent workplace/domestic violence. The implication of nursing homes being considered a home for the residents, and at the same time a workplace for staff, has psychosocial implications demanding a holistic review by care providers.

In nursing homes, some negative outcomes that fall under resident "abuse and neglect" must be investigated and reported to authorities under the industry's guidelines. In the United States, a listing of signs, types, and the definition of resident abuse, neglect, and rights in nursing homes are also available in most of the CMS-related literature, requiring care providers, residents, and families to work together to protect everyone from physical or emotional harm.

It is noteworthy that the first order of business for a holistic nursing home management is for the leadership to create a congenial living and working environment that is based on how families, residents, and staff themselves feel about issues of safety, security, rights, and freedom. Not fulfilling safety and security requests of the residents and their families, or providing adequate information if the request isn't in the best interest of the resident, is a breach of the holistic nursing home management principle.

Derlega and Janda (1981, 16) stated that "safety needs include freedom from physical harm such as the need to be protected from injury or physical abuse . . . adult must provide children with feelings of safety and security." Contextually, *children* implies the weak and the vulnerable, including those who, through diminution in health or aging process, are likely to exhibit childlike behaviors such as dependency, similar to those found among nursing home residents. Such dependencies must be recognized well documented and protected in all civilized societies.

In much the same vein, Golbert and Shostek (2007, 18–20) stated that "the promotion of resident and staff safety and an adherence to federal regulation . . . indeed safety is the number one priority even at the expense of production or efficiency." Accordingly, in nursing homes, "production or efficiency" may imply having a comprehensive risk management program.

The advocacy for a comprehensive assessment and care plan for resident safety and security needs improvement. At the lower levels of the nursing home organization, there is an urgent need for staff to conceptualize and practice how the sum of all parts for safety, security, and rights domains are connected as one whole to enhance a holistic nursing home care for residents. A comprehensive risk management program in nursing homes, therefore, is a written document that describes facility policies and protocols relative to the prevention of resident abuse and neglect, staff and public safety, physical environment safety, committee on safety, data collection, record keeping, staff behavior and training that are current, proactive, and preventive.

A nursing home's risk management program should have four broad areas as key for continuous risk management, subject to inspection; namely, resident safety, staff safety, environmental safety, and corrective actions. Even though these safety domains are monitored by different government agencies, they must be managed holistically by care providers, not only to comply with state and federal regulations, but most importantly, to provide peace of mind and a feeling of well-being for all stakeholders.

From the holistic nursing home management viewpoint, it is the inconsistency in managing resident safety and security that produces negative opinions and emotions from residents and families, affecting nursing home quality and staff morale. Most nursing home staff want to keep their residents satisfied to prevent residents' and families' complaints. However, human emotions within a state of well-being need constant nurturing since the degree of that well-being is directly proportional to the amount of safety and security available in time and place. It is important to also note that the positive emotions from residents and families are generated when they can believe and the nursing home can prove that all safety, security, and resident rights precautions are complete, functional, and that staff are well trained to successfully carry out life-safety plans in an emergency.

The impact of resident safety and security on nursing home quality is overwhelming. The implementation of holistic nursing home management is significant in helping to change the negative opinion and lack of public trust concerning resident safety and security in nursing homes. Consequently, care provers are advised to continually assess what impact the resident environment has on resident quality of life and the rating on nursing home quality. In an article titled "At Least Mom Will Be There: The Role of Resident Safety in Nursing Home Quality," Kapp (2003, 1) confirmed some of these lingering negative opinions about resident safety in nursing homes, and stated that "when family members admit a loved one to a new nursing home, they expect that the facility will assure the physical safety of the residents. However, this does not always occur."

Because this pessimistic view of nursing home care is linked to safety and security, dating back to almshouses and has continued unabated despite piles of government regulations aimed at nursing home quality, the answer to achieving nursing home quality may not lie on the regulations alone but on the management approach, leadership, staff supervision, and educational orientation inside nursing homes. Thus far, knowledge about the holistic nature of nursing home care management has been too restrictive, limiting it only as a clinical operation. An expansive knowledge is needed that is based on the concept of holistic health management and the realities of care assessment outcomes to properly manage stakeholders' expectations. However, according to OBRA '87, it is important to note that there are times when a resident's adverse event is "unavoidable," and if there is deviation in the stakeholder's expectations, it does not necessarily imply that the nursing home has been negligent. It may suggest a failure in communication and documentation before the adverse event. Therefore, it is highly recommended that caregivers in nursing homes maintain an effective line of communication between them, care recipients, and care recipients' representatives to clarify expectations in care and caring. An effective documentation is also essential as proof that adequate care was provided and received despite the adverse event.

Understanding Resident Environmental Factors Affecting Residents' Needs Satisfaction in the Holistic Health Management Perspective

Resident environment in nursing homes is defined as a conglomerate of multifaceted factors and activities contributing to the resident's well-being, holistically spanning throughout several clinical and non-clinical disciplines. Some of these factors are listed in the succeeding pages of this book denoting holistic health management as a principle of connecting all the dots in nursing home caregiving.

Resident environment also can be classified as motivating or unmotivating, bringing into focus the quality of life issues and the concept of the resident's self-determination. The responsibility of creating a motivating living environment for residents in nursing homes rests on staff treatment of residents. Human beings, in general, must be provided with certain basic psychosocial needs in order for them to survive well in their environment. Nursing homes present a unique residential environment for those who require constant care and caring with adequate support systems.

A motivating nursing home environment is one where caregivers are required to care for their residents above and beyond their call of duty. OBRA '87, states that "residents admitted into nursing homes must receive and the facility must provide services to obtain or maintain well-being." An unmotivating nursing home environment, on the other hand, is one where staff/resident interaction is poor, where residents are not treated with respect and dignity, and where the physical environment is not conducive to residents' overall well-being. Creating a motivating nursing home environment, which is responsibility of nursing management and staff, begins with safety and security for the residents.

Behavior theorists have attributed man's psychosocial maladjustment—such as phobias, hysteria, anxiety, depression, and other forms of neurosis—to his unfavorable environmental conditions. Human beings have the tendency to adjust well, to live normal lives in societies or conditions that are organized with the designs for safety and security.

According to Derlega and Janda (1981, 17), "Neurotic depression is usually brought about by an event that would make anyone feel sad and unhappy." Liebert and Spiegler (1974, 103) defined neurosis "as a psychological disorder characterized by much anxiety with which the person has difficulty coping and by abnormal behavior such as irrational fear (phobias), obsessional thoughts and as in hysteria, physical complaints." Accordingly, there are countless health implications to humans, especially for nursing home residents, who live in or experience unsafe and dehumanizing living conditions. According to the Code of Federal Register (CFR) for nursing homes, however, there is a basic prerequisite toward nursing hone quality for safety, which is that "the facility must provide a safe, functional, sanitary, and comfortable environment for residents, staff and the public" (Pate and yale, 2009, CFR 483.70(h) F465)

A hazard-free environment relates to the physical plant configurations, resident supervision, and general plan of care suitable for the sick and frail individuals who can no longer age in place or survive independently in the community. The Americans with Disability Act of 1900 (ADA) has acted as a watchdog to protect disabled individuals from discrimination, direct neglect, and direct threat, defining "threat as a significant risk to health or safety of others that cannot be eliminated by reasonable accommodation." Most nursing homes are designed to meet ADA specification and standards, and are scrutinized at least once a year by the designated law enforcement agency for continued compliance.

In 1954, Abraham Maslow theorized his hierarchy of human needs beginning with the physiological need for safety. According to the hierarchical design and interpretation of the needs theory, belongingness, esteem, and lastly, self-actualization will not be achieved if safety needs are not met. It is noteworthy to care providers that nursing home residents must first feel safe and secure in order for them to be able to benefit from their wellness programs.

Accordingly, Maslow divided human needs into two groups; namely, the basic needs and the mega needs. Basic needs are physiological, safety and security, while higher level needs are half of belongingness, esteem, and self-actualization. Maslow then draws a distinction in human needs and the impact each group of needs would have on the deprived individual. In a book titled *Motivation: Theory and Research*, Cofer and Appley (1967, 676) defined mega human needs as "instinctoid," meaning that "many of them especially the higher ones are not strong enough to be apparent unless conditions favor their manifestation."

Safety and security precautions designed to prevent humans from physical or emotional harm are basic needs. If basic needs are not provided, their strong "manifestations" will trigger maladjustments in humans, especially in the young, the frail, and the elderly. Safety and the avoidance of pain are related concepts that must be clearly understood by care providers with regards to care and caring for the elderly. It is normal for human beings to seek to withdraw from painful stimuli and to avoid objects that bring them pain and discomfort. Nursing homes should be managed to bring comfort and joy to the residents.

It is important to note that human beings who are strong and healthy can fend for themselves when their health, safety, and security are threatened. The opposite is true of the young, the frail, and the elderly, who oftentimes depend on the action of others for protection.

In 2001, the District of Columbia Municipal Regulation (DCMR) provided a list of sentinel events to include pain, pressure ulcer, restraint, depression, dehydration, and constipation. Sentinel health events are defined as "one that guards or warns of approaching danger" (*Webster's II New Riverside Dictionary*, 1996, 619), demanding a careful and immediate medical response by health care providers and plan of care. Resident fall is another high-risk factor for resident safety, seconded by elopement for the elderly in nursing homes. Even though resident falls and elopement risks are not officially listed as sentinel health events, they nevertheless need to be taken seriously, with careful residents' assessments, plans of care, and follow-ups.

With regards to careful planning for falls to avoid negligence claims, Dewitt (2007, 24) wrote:

> *Even residents with normal balance and gait and who do not take medication affecting blood pressure or sensorium may trip and fall in a facility. A single fall is isolated and is not generally grounds for negligence but residents who require eyeglasses or who use assistive devices for ambulation present a higher degree of risk for falls and require careful scrutiny.*

We advocate that care providers in nursing homes using holistic health management approach to provide residents' needs hierarchically upward, starting with physiological needs for safety and security. Rakich, Longest, and Darr (1977, 341) stated that "once the survival needs are met, attention can be turned to ensuring continued survival by protection of oneself against physical harm and deprivation." Failure to provide residents with human needs in the ascending order of needs will prevent them from achieving higher needs. They can be traumatized to exhibit behavior conditions, which Karen Horney calls neurotic needs.

Cafer and Appley (1967, 630) cited Horney as a student of Sigmund Freud who confirmed that "feelings of insecurity may give rise to basic anxiety" in humans, causing them to develop strategies in an attempt to cope with these untenable feelings. Such strategies Horney calls "neurotic needs" because they are often "irrational." Smith and Smith (1958, 463) defined neurosis within the context of basic need deprivation "as a sustained patterning of reaction involving anxiety, fear and endless trouble that pervades significant aspects of an individual's life." Coleman (1972, 218), in the same vein, described "a neurotic behavior as a circular process in which an individual has basic feelings of inadequacy and inferiority which leads to the evaluation of everyday problems as threatening and to the resultant arousal of anxiety."

It is unclear how much of the neurotic needs such as depression found among the elderly in nursing homes are community or facility acquired. However, Rosen (2007, 26) asserted that "approximately 15% of nursing home residents experience major depression and an additional 25% complain of significant depressive symptoms."

Lack of safety measures for the elderly in nursing homes can also manifest in residents when they exhibit a withdraw symptom for activities (abilities) of daily living (ADLs), such as scheduled showers, because of prior experience with inadequate water temperatures. Residents can even develop incontinency due to irrational fear of falling based on the resident's prior experience of falls.

There are also rampant reported cases of theft in nursing homes involving residents' valuables that leave them vulnerable, fearful, and distrustful of their nursing home domicile and staff. Long-term care law requires safe and secure spaces for residents' valuables. Per regulation, an investigation must be conducted when a theft or loss of resident property occurs, but due to declined cognitive abilities or memory loss of residents, no eyewitness, or uncooperative staff behaviors, the investigation may be inconclusive. However, whenever theft of a resident's valuables occur, it causes residents' psychological trauma and "a feeling of insecurity causing them pain and a reduction in the quality of life" (Umoren 1992, 665).

Another example of a traumatic situation would be one in which a resident was on a psych-medication for manic depressive disorder. The resident stopped taking the medication for five years and functioned well in the community until her nursing home placement, when her manic-depressive disorder resumed. Based on this example, care providers are encouraged to avoid any situational or environmental factors that are high in "triggering abnormal behavior in nursing home residents. We advise that new residents who have been assessed and admitted into nursing homes receive initial close monitoring by both care providers and families to ensure that residents are psychosocially well adjusted to their new environment.

Most nursing home residents who develop psychosocial disorders may be referred to the psychiatrists for medications. Some of these abnormal behaviors can easily be traced to environmental factors or staff behavior. Psychiatric referrals should be applied as the last resort after all situational/ environmental implications have been cleared.

It should be noted that physical and chemical restraints in nursing homes are against federal and state Laws unless they are justified, and that sufficient efforts have been demonstrated and documented by nursing homes to reduce them. Accordingly, the IDT (interdisciplinary team) must adequately assess residents periodically for nonpharmaceutical interventions and to prevent labeling residents as "noncompliant" when they may be needing different plans of care more appropriate to them. ORBA '87 (Omnibus Budget Reconciliation Act), which is an act of United States Congress, has demanded that "the facility must develop a comprehensive care plan for each resident that includes measurable objectives and timetables to meet a resident's medical, nursing, and mental and psychosocial needs that are identified in the comprehensive assessment" (OBRA '87, CFR 483.20 p.279).

Protecting nursing home residents from physical or emotional harm is an important consideration under OBRA '87 and OBRA '90. Providing safety and security for residents with mental illness is hereby recognized as a difficult 24/7 job for care providers, and is noted to be a big part in measuring nursing home quality as well as meeting LTC guidelines for compliance.

The inability of nursing homes to totally meet these guidelines, which are tailored toward resident-need satisfaction for safety, is still acutely felt today, predating OBRA '87. Consequently, state and federal surveyors are tightening their surveillance activities to ensure that the nursing home environment is safe and humane for the residents. They believe that nursing homes must uphold high standards for resident safety and security, and must be held accountable as more disabled people are entering nursing homes. Statistics show that the reasons given for residents being admitted into nursing homes are related to their age-related declines in ADLs, disease process, or post medical surgeries. Hooyman and Kijak (1988, 359-360) pointed out that:

> *Approximately 80% of all people over 65 will spend some time in a nursing home at some point during later life . . . Although the majority of nursing home residents are functionally impaired and unable to live independently in the Community it is noteworthy that for every impaired older person in the long term care facility, there are two and perhaps as many as five equally impaired older person residing in the community.*

Colbert (2007, 54) disagreed that the nursing home is for older people alone, and posited "we think nursing homes are just for old people but that's not always true. Nursing homes also exist for people like me. Most people in nursing homes are old, but it isn't age that gets them there. It is disabilities, the kind that make us unable to get in and out of bed or get dressed or go to the bathroom on our own." Accordingly, we expect future numbers of nursing home admissions to rise in response to more baby boomers entering the golden age, and because of the greater number of disabled individuals who still live in the community. This assessment is in contrast to Anderson (2007,92), who has predicted a continuous decline in nursing home use between 2006 and 2030, and pointed out that "nursing home use by 'oldest' old or those aged 85 and older has declined sharply since 1984."

As can be expected, and as an update to care providers, residents entering nursing homes do so with limited abilities to observe safety and security rules on their own, making them partially or completely dependent on others for protection. Most residents are injury-prone, especially to falls, due to diminution in health status or youthfulness. In an article titled "Don't Forget Why You're Here," O'Connor (2006, 18) argued that when families entrust their loved ones into nursing homes for various reasons, to include respite care, "they want to be able to trust you . . . but like desert survival rules, they can be fatal if ignored."

Resident safety and security has remained the number one primary concern for families and lawmakers. Their escalating disgust and mistrust for nursing homes are well documented to include threats of litigation. Care providers must adjust nursing home quality to being heavily weighted toward safety and security concerns. Nursing homes must ensure their quality assurance capabilities to produce positive safety outcomes for the residents. They must demonstrate their abilities, above all else, to protect residents in order for them to be in good standing with millions of stakeholders who may already have some axe to grind with nursing homes.

In an article titled "Double Blind," Fleck (2006, 18) observed that currently "more than 44 million Americans are involved in caring for an aging relative or friend." In an article titled "Nursing Homes: A Citizen's Action Guide," Horn and Griesel (1977, 3) analyzed residential experience in nursing homes and wrote that "nursing homes are more capable of striking fear, anxiety, and despair among the old." In another article, titled "Residents Say Quality of Life Is lacking in Long-Term Care Setting," Powilis (1990, 12–20) observed that "residents' lives in nursing homes are boring and monotonous . . ."

Care providers in nursing homes have the responsibility not only to strive toward consumer satisfaction but to help alleviate working families from fear that their loved ones are not safe and secure in nursing homes. It is noteworthy that families who place their loved ones in nursing homes expect nursing homes to provide a safer, more stable, and a more secure environment where the prevalence of accidental patient injuries would be minimized or nonexistent, and that "residents' abilities of daily living do not diminish unless . . . diminution was unavoidable" (Facility Guide to OBRA Regulation, Interpretive Guidelines . . . 2001, 84).

Patient negative outcomes (injuries) leading to actual physical harm to the resident are oftentimes classified as poor "quality of care" issues (OBRA '87, CFR483.25, F 309). These resident-negative care outcomes exist in different forms, such as falls with fractures, medication errors, elopement, fires, food poisoning, wounds, and lack of freedom from physical or chemical restraints. Patient-negative care outcomes in the psychosocial-emotive perspective are also important and were partially discussed in the previous pages.

On the other hand, how well or how poorly residents in nursing homes are treated vis-à-vis resident rights, abuse, and dignity as they interact with staff and families is classified as "quality of life" issues. Specifically, "a facility must care for its residents in a manner and in an environment that promotes maintenance or enhancement of each resident's quality of life . . . dignity and respect in full recognition of his or her individuality" (OBRA '87, CFR 483.15, 15Af-240–250).

Chapter 9

Factors of Responsibility and Accountability in Holistic Management in Nursing Homes

There are many written and unwritten action plans under the banner of holding nursing homes responsible and accountable for failure to meet regulatory standards. Written expectations are those expectations for compliance found in federal, state, and municipal regulations. The unwritten expectations are those expectations held by residents' families and loved ones, which may be objective or subjective. Nevertheless, they should never be overlooked.

An example of an intersection of the written and unwritten expectations can be found when a resident's representative walks into a resident's room unannounced and finds the resident lying in a pool of urine despite the written expectation that bedridden residents be checked X number of times by staff to prevent wetness and the eventual development of pressure ulcers. This breach in expectations allows the representative to file a complaint with the facility administrator or with the State Board Agency and the Nursing Home Ombudsman Agency (NHOA), a.k.a. Long-Term Care Ombudsman Program (LTCOP), for remedy. The ombudsman, which is a Swedish word meaning "advocate," was formed in the United States in 1981. In nursing homes, the function of the ombudsman, working hand in hand with other state agencies, is to advocate for resident rights for quality of life, quality of care, resident environment, resident fund management, and most importantly, equity in resident admissions, transfer, and discharge. The ombudsman must have access to the facility 24/7.

We have already emphasized the seriousness of resident safety and security. Nursing homes are expected to immediately report to their state regulatory authorities anything or a situation that threatens the health, safety, and security of each resident, and to make corrections that demonstrate a proactive and preventive approach. Nursing home administrators are required to uphold ethical standards that are issued to them alongside their administrator's license to practice. Violations of safety or administrative code conduct that cause resident's physical and emotional harm (potential or actual) are the leading cause of heavy penalties within the long-term care enforcement grid, supported by reasons for nursing homes being so heavily regulated to protect residents from harm. McPherson (2000, 1) wrote: "notification regarding incidents can be received on the hotline . . . all telephone incidents must be followed with a written notification within 24 hours or the next workday." Accordingly, in 2001, District of Columbia Municipal Regulations (DCMR) mandated that "Each incident shall be documented in the resident's record and report to the Licensing Agency within forty eight (48) hours of occurrence except that incidents and accidents that result in harm to the resident shall be reported to the Licensing Agency within eight (8) hours of occurrence" (DCMR 3232.4, 37 DCR 3394, p. 31). The Code of Federal Register (CFR) and OBRA '87 483.25, F-309 mandate that in a nursing home, "each resident must receive the care and services to attain or maintain the highest practicable physical, mental and psychosocial wellbeing in accordance with the comprehensive assessment and plan of care" (Facility Guide to OBRA Regulations, Interpretive Guidelines . . . (2009).

Confounded and overwhelmed by public expectations, innumerable regulatory demands, the proverbial truth about residents' preexisting health conditions, the mythical guarantee for resident safety, the demand for zero tolerance for residents' negative health outcome or injuries under the banner of regulatory safety violations, the disregard for residents' age-related health problems, disease process, and residents' limited physical and mental abilities, some nursing homes are becoming targets for trial lawyers. It is also possible for caregivers to feel unworthy and become desensitized as nursing home quality is constantly characterized as substandard. Most stakeholders have these unwritten expectations responsible for provoking strong emotions whenever a negative resident care outcome, such as resident falls, occur and are reported. Resident falls are the most prevalent, most documented resident incident in nursing homes, and perhaps the most worrisome to families. Frequent resident falls and other resident incidents in nursing homes are usually reviewed by the state licensing agency, who may sanction the nursing home based on resident incident prevention and resident supervision. The public's decry of nursing homes' effectiveness in preventing residents' incidents, preventable or not, may add to the waning trust between nursing homes and stakeholders, and a rush to judgement.

Trust and empathy can be a bilateral venture, a two-way street between nursing homes, families, and other stakeholders. Nursing home staffers, knowing that it is never an easy decision for a family member to admit another family member into a nursing home, are expected to express due diligence in caregiving. Before the family decides to admit a loved one in a nursing home, there is usually a fair amount of introspection, followed by a gradual development of trust in the care provider. We expect the families/stakeholders likewise to learn patience in understanding the difficulty involved in taking care of an adult person in an institution perhaps he/she never anticipated.Because we know that the request to have mutual trust and understanding can be an important but not easy an achievement, there is a need for nursing home leadership to invest a sufficient amount of time and effort to educate staff, stakeholders, and families on residents' susceptibilities to maintain the trust and the credibility they need to overcome the public perception of nursing homes as the modern-day poorhouses. Oftentimes, we hear of resident neglect and abuse in nursing homes, some of which have made newspaper headlines, such as "an employee of a nursing home in Monroe, Michigan, was charged with neglect of an adult resident allegedly leading to the resident's death . . . the nursing facility's administrator and director of nursing were also charged for failing to report the incident to authorities as required by law" (*Long-Term Care Interface*, 2006, 42).

Resident safety and security are the quickest ways for the public at large to evaluate, document, and hold nursing homes accountable for lack of nursing home quality. Nursing homes, therefore, through daily and individual resident assessments, must protect them from harm, bottom line. Dewitt (2007, 24) shed a new and optimistic light on the future performances of nursing homes, and stated that "Most providers are eager to improve the quality of care provided to residents and to increase consumer satisfaction as much as possible." Additionally, we strongly believe that under a holistic management approach, a fair amount of the contributing factors to an unsafe and unsecure nursing home environment for residents are amendable when resident/staff ratios are small, when staff are properly trained, when staff are effectively supervised and held accountable on their job responsibilities.

Consequently, staff must learn to complete their comprehensive incident reports (CIR) promptly, accurately, and meaningfully, especially the column marked "Intervention," denoting how they hope to prevent future occurrences. For an example, in one nursing home, a CIR was completed for a demented resident who often wandered around and assaulted other residents. This resident's intervention on the CIR was to have a sitter 24/7. On this day, this resident did have a sitter, so he/she wandered into another resident's room. A fight ensued and he/she was badly beaten up, with injury to the forehead. In completing the CIR meaningfully and as part of ensuring a comprehensive investigation, staff must carefully examine/ assess the resident's cognitive abilities and staff supervision for causations.

Another important part of safety promotions and injuries prevention for residents in nursing homes is the extent to which higher management of the organization is involved in supporting safety promotion and safety maintenance to prevent resident injuries that seem to plague nursing homes, portraying them in a negative light to the public. Most recent surveys of the American health care services have ranked nursing homes at the bottom. In an article titled "It's All about Change," Benner (2006, 10) wrote that "nurses are ranked first at 89%, doctors at 69%, hospitals at 64%, drug companies at 43%, nursing homes at 35%, Insurance Companies at 34%, and lastly HMOs at 30%."

For years, nursing home administrators and their governing boards have tried in vain to explain or correct their dismal performance report card, which most often than not is caused by related resident safety and security issues. It is important that residents' safety and security in nursing homes are not violated. Equally important is that each negative outcome be thoroughly, professionally, fairly investigated, needing a collaborative understanding between care providers and stakeholders as nursing homes are transitioning themselves to meet public expectations. Collaborative action means empathy and not sympathy from the public, and the regulatory agencies to realistically evaluate nursing home quality beyond the current stringent regulations.

To fully understand geriatric care at the emotional level, sympathy denotes "a feeling or expression of sorrow for another's distress or loss," while empathy is "identification with an understanding of the thoughts or feelings of another" (*Webster's II, New Riverside Dictionary*, 1996, 227–684). Empathy, not sympathy, is needed in defining what achieving quality in nursing homes means so that stakeholders and care providers can meaningfully interface and coordinate their expectations.

With regards to care providers' and stakeholders' actions, what specific areas of collaboration exist? Both must learn more about the process of normal aging as it affects the biological and psychological functioning in humans, which is hoped to create a zone of mutual acceptance regarding status change in the elderly in nursing homes. For the oldest old and their negative health outcomes, whether in nursing homes or in the community, the controversy lies in locating the blurred intersection or separation point between nature and nurture.

Other areas needing mutual understanding are found in reviewing some long-term care laws and residents' health status, such as resident rights, resident autonomy, the disease process such as Alzheimer's, dementia, psychosis, and osteoporosis, as they impact resident safety beyond the control of even the most conscientious care provider.We need to further seek an understanding of the relative impact of the limited resources to provide an ideal staffing ratio/resident supervision for almost 90 percent of the resident population in the nursing home who are already susceptible to falls. There is also the inability of care providers to provide a balanced response to residents with physical/mental limitations but with the desire to exercise their primordial rights for autonomy and independence. It is like expecting a miracle. With these controversies still intact, it is possible for the nursing home quality and public opinion polls to remain unacceptably low for the foreseeable future.

In the main, are resident negative outcomes (injuries) in nursing homes preventable? This question, when closely examined, is intended to bring stakeholders face-to-face with care providers on the reality of caring for an elderly individual with multiple chronic debilitating diseases, who on one hand are very much loved by close relatives and families, but on the other hand have posed significant challenges even to most compassionate rank-and-file care providers. Nevertheless, given the current government mandates and stakeholder concerns for resident safety, nursing homes must update their facility policies and practices and staff training relative to resident health, safety, and security. They must understand that the enforcement grid and the public opinion are interpreted based on how many resident injuries or abuse occur in nursing homes due to safety violations.

The content of all the federal K- and F-tags under OBRA '87 and OBRA '90, not including state statutes, should be studied and analyzed with emphasis on resident safety and security, which is interpreted to mean residents' comfort and well-being without adverse events. The dichotomy existing between the possibility of achieving an ideal nursing home quality and avoidance of residents' negative outcome having either actual or potential immediate jeopardy to residents require an empirical study. Nursing homes are held accountable for poor care performance in various ways to include an ongoing civil monetary penalty until the infraction is resolved, a declaration of a focus facility status (FFS), denial of new admissions, and closure of the facility.

There is a direct correlation between the degree of harm from resident-negative outcome and the gravity of penalties. The deficiency scores a nursing home receives are issued with the scope and severity (S & S) on the enforcement grid. Accordingly, nursing home deficiencies are cited by regulatory enforcement in the descending order of A to L on the S & S enforcement grid. Each letter represents the likelihood that the infraction on the statute had caused actual harm or had the potential to cause emotional or physical harm to the resident. For example, a resident elopement or a resident fall with a fracture could get a facility a G on the S & S enforcement grid. We do not mean to imply that this is the only reason for receiving a bad score on the S & S enforcement grid. There could be other reasons, such as repeat deficiencies, the overall facility practices, the track records of the nursing home as identified in OSCAR (online survey, certification, and reports), and the human factor of the law enforcement agent. Specifically, the scope and severity assigned to nursing home infractions is based on the "degree of harm (actual or potential) related to the non-compliance" (Pate and Yale, 2005, 327). Government inspections conducted annually at a minimum are to "ensure that the nursing home residents receive quality care and services in a safe and comfortable environment in accordance with rules established by CMS.

Resident safety and security in nursing homes must therefore become the number one concern for continued quality assurance and performance improvement in all nursing homes seeking survival. To this end, nursing homes must be willing to accept the responsibility when resident safety problems arise in the facility. In some measures, safety violations can be caused by inanimate objects in the environment, but on the whole, it is the staff/care providers' behavior problems, ranging from ill-conceived facility policies and practices, to poor building construction, cluttered living environments, and lack of staff training and resident supervision relative to safety standards and health promotions. Most importantly, nursing homes are encouraged to resist the use of impersonal terms as "accidents" or "incidents" to describe resident-negative outcomes instead of the term "loss control" to describe their safety violations.

The concept of loss control has a psychosocial meaning denoting that whenever there is an adverse event, it is caused by a human being who deviated from the norm. The fact remains, safety standards in nursing homes are upheld or not upheld by human beings who can be held accountable for infractions or be trained or retrained to achieve safety goals set by the facility. Incidents or accidents are defined conceptually as "act of God" or "natural disasters" because they are caused by providence alone; meaning something was meant to happen and nothing could be done to prevent it. With the concept of loss control defined, a high percentage of safety and security problems in nursing homes can be traceable to human errors in various forms. It further affirms that most resident injuries are preventable and that remedial actions to prevent them are achievable.

In an article titled "One-Third of Skilled Nursing Patients Harmed in Treatment," Allen (2014) conducted a study that revealed nearly 22,000 patient monthly injuries, of which over 1,500 of them died, adding that "doctors who reviewed the patients' records determined that 59 percent of the errors and injuries were preventable" (Wikipedia 2020, para 3). However, in all human endeavors, mistakes can be made, even with the best intentions, as long as we learn from them to avoid repetition.

The history of spaceflights and their early incidents/accidents come as a reminder that adverse events that are not caused by providence can be investigated and fixed. Staff in nursing homes must be taught to accept mistakes when they occur so that teaching and learning can take place to prevent further safety violations in the future. Most importantly, there has to exist a higher level of consciousness of the pain and suffering, even death, caused to a resident due to a preventable human error.

In a book titled *Industrial Psychology*, McCormick and Tiffin (1974, 510) discussed the cause of industrial accidents and the negative outcomes of safety violations, and stated that "we sometimes think of accidents as events that 'just happen,' but in our more rational moments we should of course realize that they really are brought about by some combination of present circumstances and preceding events."

By making human behavior (behavior modification) the centerpiece of maintaining resident safety and security compliance with the LTC regulations to protect residents from harm, nursing homes can move much closer to achieving nursing home quality. We find issues relating to resident safety and security as forming the main source of complaints from families and regulatory enforcement. Nursing homes must routinely assess to identify vulnerable residents to assure adequate supervision, teach safety promotion and injury prevention techniques to staff, provide adequate supervision to direct care staff, and to evaluate their actions through legal and regulatory lenses to ensure that each care they give to residents meets safety and security standards.

Chapter 10

Other Related Care Areas in the Holistic Management of Nursing Homes: Resident Care and the Environment

There are two broad implications that can be deduced from the phrase "homelike environment" in nursing homes as contained in CFR 483.10(1) F-584 that every administrator should be aware of. Psychosocially, the nursing home environment should make residents feel better, not worse, about themselves. Environmentally, it should be clean, sanitary, safe, and with necessary amenities that deemphasize as much as possible the institutional aspects of the current nursing homes.

Let's start with the physical plant as it relates to the resident live-in environment. Under the holistic nursing home management, the relationship between the resident live-in environment and his quality of life cannot be overemphasized. The physical environment should be created not only to provide personal comfort for the residents but also to provide the first impression suggestive of the quality of care they are likely to receive. Most residents or their representatives as customers have used their initial tour of the facility to make their decisions to accept or reject their residency. Among other things, a resident's decision to choose or not to choose a particular nursing home as a dwelling place may be based on the problem of odor, cleanliness, staff behavior toward residents, resident behavior toward other residents, its general appearance. We have chosen to repeat these points as they are likely to have a negative impact on resident admissions and the survival of the particular nursing home as a business institution. Becoming a holistic nursing home administrator demands that the administrator and managers of nursing homes to be intrusively involved in all aspects of resident care in order to fully understand and master what the term "resident environment" means. While the term "resident environment" in and of itself is not new, the right interpretation of its meaning and its application have been unbelievably small. What comes to mind is making frequent environmental rounds, visiting and getting to meet and know the residents in their living quarters, asking them questions about their care, assessing and assuring the physical plant compliance, and participating in clinical assessments of resident health conditions, with the goal of creating a total well-being for the resident and staff education as needed. The administrator and the managers will at this point be able to develop a preventive or proactive approach to customer service and toward appropriate care for the residents. If administrators are able to perceive residents and their environment in the same empathetic and emotional lens as the family/resident representative do, they will be able to develop an effective facility preventive program needed to address the frequently reported family concerns, which include those we are enunciating below under the headings of sentinel events, prevention of sentinel events, signs of a poorly managed nursing home that make family members angry, and tips to an interdisciplinary approach to preventing offensive odors in nursing homes.

These are issues that generally relate to the residents' quality of life and their environment. They are issues that are immediately linked to the facility's face validity and the doom and gloom of the nursing home in general, impinging on our sense of humanity for the helpless. Families of the residents are usually angry, for example, when they see their loved ones soaked in urine, smell of urine, find them untidy or their general living conditions deplorable. Blanchard (2016), in an article titled "6 Signs of Nursing Home Neglect," cited some nursing home red flags/issues for which families should notify the local ombudsman as follows, "poor personal hygiene, unsanitary living conditions, physical issues from lack of nutrition, loss or lack of mobility, unexplained injuries and psychological issues" (Wikipedia, 2019, para 1–4).

Making daily environmental rounds, visiting residents, and conducting clinical reviews therefore should be done, not only with the mindset of looking for these red flags but also for an opportunity for a holistic-minded administrator to ask himself the basic question, "Can I live under this condition in which I find my residence?" This is an insinuating question to which the nursing home administrator's answer is intended to be based on either the interpretive guidelines of OBRA '87, personal empathy, or countertransference, requiring a call an immediate corrective action if what he sees or feels reflects substandard care.

Accordingly, we recommend that the administrative functions of the holistic nursing home administrators include their ability to utilize their sense of touch, smell, taste, hearing, and sight to empirically collect the data they will need to develop effective preventive programs and staff training.

Facility-specific empirical evidence of negative implications to care that is personally collected by the administrators or their agents is likely to be more useful in developing preventive programs. Fall prevention, pressure-ulcer prevention, incontinency prevention, odor prevention are a few health-related conditions where personal knowledge of each resident is better than any information derived from secondary sources. It is noteworthy to apply the meaning of empirical knowledge that states "by seeing, hearing, smelling, feeling, and tasting, we form our conception of the world around us" (Kneller 1971, 215).

Our experience shows that the first step to achieving customer satisfaction is giving customers what they want or giving or doing something to someone they would not give or do to themselves. Beyond the regulatory mandates, nursing home quality begins when employees start "putting themselves in the shoes of their residents." There are many employees who are already dedicated in doing this, but there could be much more. Seeking customer satisfaction is the standard of practice that applies to any business enterprise that seeks survival. In nursing homes, creating preventive programs in areas of service is to believe in the old adage that "prevention is better than cure." According to OBRA '87, it is stated that a resident admitted into a nursing home "must receive and the facility must provide the necessary care and services to attain or maintain the highest practicable physical, mental, and psycho-social well-being in accordance with the comprehensive assessment and plan of care (OBRA Interpretive Guidelines, 1987).

Consequently, we have identified four broad areas essential in nursing homes for which undivided attention, knowledge, and prevention by the holistic nursing home administrators and staffers are needed. They are listed as follows:

Sentinel/adverse events in nursing homes

- New fractures/falls
- Patient behaviors affecting others (lack of staff supervision)
- Patient depression
- Nine or more medications
- Fecal impaction
- Urinary tract infection without catheter use
- Weight loss/gain (needs close examination of causation)
- Restraints
- Dehydration
- Unexplained declined in patient health condition
- Pressure ulcers
- Pain
- Patient elopement
- Shortage of trained nursing staff

Prevention of sentinel/adverse events

- Identify and develop a specific policy and procedure for each sentinel event
- Train staff to follow policies and procedures when caring for patients
- Monitor care "hierarchically" to ensure that facility policies and procedures are followed by every caregiver

- Assure adequate recordkeeping and documentation, which includes tracking and trending
- Report resident incident timely to the DON, administrator, attending physician unto the DOH
- Train staff on the legal and regulatory implications of incidence of adverse preventable events
- Train staff to routinely ask patients questions relating to each area of the sentinel event; findings must be reported immediately to a clinical supervisor unto the attending physician for immediate corrective action
- Document all activities relating to sentinel events in the clinical record
- Ensure a consistent staff assignment to each patient as much as practicable
- Conduct a "hierarchical" patient clinical assessment on admission and ongoing
- Care plan resident care with empathy
- Provide enough staff with supervision

Signs of Poorly Managed Nursing Homes: Family and Resident Concerns

- Not enough meaningful resident therapeutic activities, especially for bedridden residents who are lonely, bored, and needing more than BESM (bingo, eat, sleep, and medication)
- Unkempt residents for grooming, odor of the mouth, body, and clothing
- Urine smells (not fecal) on resident and in the room
- Staff talking too loudly in care areas (congregating and doing nothing)
- Staff being rude and rough with residents
- Staff personal hygiene and body odor
- Staff professional appearance without name tags
- Staff unfriendly communication or no meaningful communication with residents

- Staff unfriendly/wrong communication with family members (staff professional attitudes stink)
- Resident drooling without staff attention
- Poor tasting, looking, cold foods (overall dining arrangement)
- Missing resident personal belongings without investigation and redress
- Dirty and cluttered resident rooms and facility
- Incompatible roommates
- Strong urine odors, fecal stain on resident or furniture, room clutter and untidiness
- Staff not using dominant language in care areas or not mindful of resident presence
- Staff delays in or not answering resident call (bell) for help
- Staff are not empathetic toward the resident (please note that residents need your empathy, not sympathy)
- Staff not assisting resident during meals
- Poor room temperatures and ventilation
- Staff not knocking on door each time before entering resident room and not identifying himself/herself to the resident
- Deprivation of resident sleep and rest because of noise level
- Rampant reports/rumors of resident abuse and neglect/frequent resident falls/pressure ulcers/not enough staff
- Uncontrolled behavior of residents detrimental to other residents
- Resident has contraction, skin tear, weight loss, pressure ulcer, etc. without sufficient explanation or family notification since last visit (note resident significant change)
- Staff using or answering personal cellphones in care areas
- Staff using profane language in care areas or in the presence of resident
- Resident left in dayrooms or nursing stations unattended
- Bad state/federal surveys
- Not enough staff
- Lack of effective communication between staff and resident/ resident representative
- Cluttered corridors, dirty and unpolished floors
- Ungroomed outside environment/yard

Prevention of Offensive Odors and Holistic Management in Nursing Homes

Offensive odors in nursing homes have negative impact on residents' quality of life, quality of care, and customer satisfaction outcomes. Most public opinions have identified nursing home odors as the number one concern. Greenberg (2016), in an article titled "Nursing Home Facilities and Housekeeping: Odor and Stain Control," wrote "in fact when visiting prospective nursing homes there is one distinct observation that can be vital in the decision making process: offensive odor" (Wikipedia 2020, para1). One mistake that has been made with respect to nursing home odor is that it is caused by the housekeeping department and they alone can correct it. Causes of nursing home odors are many, some relating to overall staff uncooperative behavior, defective cleaning technique, scheduled cleaning, and resident care plans. Resident-felt needs are identified in the care conference and monitored for change in condition. The good news is that all contributing factors to nursing home odors are preventable, demanding an interdepartmental approach from everyone—nursing, maintenance, and housekeeping—working together to:

- Identify in writing the source of odor—namely, residents with either body, urine, or fecal odors—and care plan them
- Identify in writing all incontinent residents and care plan them
- Assure that residents' scheduled showers are given and monitored for compliance
- Assure that residents' personal hygiene of the mouth, perineal are done
- Assure that proper wound care and dressing changes are done
- Ensure that the urinals and bed pans are frequently emptied and cleaned
- Identify in writing all problem resident rooms and schedule frequent maintenance for cleaning/resident care
- Assure that proper cleaning/sanitization/infection control methods with appropriate chemical solutions and measurements are followed
- Ensure that the in/out airflow ventilations are operational throughout the facility

- Remove dirty/soiled linen/personal clothing, bag them, and store in soiled utility room with doors and windows closed.
- Provide adequate staff supervision and QA at all times for numbers 1–10
- Provide adequate staff education on odor prevention tips
- Ensure foul odors are reported promptly and corrective action taken promptly

Chapter 11

Technology-Driven Health Care Delivery and Holistic Management in Nursing Homes

From the Stone Age to the Information Age, humans have been accustomed to acquiring new knowledge, leading to new discoveries in science, medicine, technology, and management. Today, there is much more discussion about telemedicine and holistic management as the new way for future health care delivery. The shared interest in telemedicine and holistic management represents an integrated health care enabling different health care providers and specialists to remotely interface with one another and share patient health information, especially on patients with disease comorbidities. Today, there exists that interdependency between medical practice and technology. So "in the healthcare industry, the dependence on medical technology cannot be overstated and as a result of the development of these brilliant inventions, healthcare practitioners can continue to find ways to improve their practice . . ." (Wikipedia 2019, para. 2).

In an article titled "The Future of Healthcare is Here: The Pandemic Has Turned Telehealth from a Maybe, One Day, to a Right Here, Right Now," Lenzer (2020, 21) wrote:

As recent as last year, only 8 percent of Americans had ever used telemedicine. That has changed overnight, with some practitioners reporting that up to 95 percent of patient visits are now "virtual," and with insurance companies and health providers advertising their telemedicine offerings

What about nursing homes? In recent years, there is a growing awareness that increased information technology and telemedicine would be advantageous in nursing home care as well, even though there are concerns whether or not nursing homes are already lagging behind. In an article titled "Building a Health Information Technology Infrastructure in Long-Term Care," Babalola et al. (2014) wrote "there is increasing interest in the potential of health information technology (HIT) to improve quality of care, prevent medical errors, and increase administrative efficiencies in the nursing home setting" (Wikipedia 2019, para.1).

Inventions with heuristic value have to be recorded and preserved to inspire future innovations, ensure improvement in technology and in continued education. Living in modern times means having the ability to use health maintenance programs and all of what modern medical technology can offer to assist human beings to live better, age better, and even live longer than their parents and grandparents.

As we have already documented, during the Industrial Revolution, modern technology was noted for bringing a speedy and efficient production in agricultural and manufacturing industries when machines were used to reduce human labor and increase the standard of living. Accordingly, the speculation that medical technologies will eliminate or reduce human labor in healthcare by automation demands further investigation.

In an article titled "Medical Automation—A Technically Enhanced Work Environment to Reduce the Burden of Care on Nursing Staff and a Solution to the Health Care Cost Crises" (Felder 2003 p S7), outlined his view and the future promise of medical automation relating to the reduction in medical errors and in the cost of healthcare. Felder conceded, however, that persons of age sixty-five and above who have ADL and quality of life needs are yet to be captured by medical technology, questioning how the ADLs in the elderly are assessed and managed, and wrote:

> *The challenges faced by our medical system are to maintain the safety, quality of life, general health, and the dignity of our elders. A high quality of life includes preserving the social group and maintaining mobility . . . and independence . . . Provide a better quality of life for our elders, we must be able to provide early predictors of the onset of chronic disease, loss of mobility, and assessment of isolation and loss of quality of life . . . There is no comprehensive tool for assessing the functional capabilities of the elder.*

Noteworthy is the school of thought with a reminder that healthcare delivery is biopsychosocial unlike other industries. Biopsychosocial health care delivery implies an appropriate interdisciplinary interaction of psychological, biological, and the socio-environmental factors to achieve wellness in patients, especially among the aged and those residing in nursing homes. We see medical technology as a useful adjunct to the humanistic approach needed in holistic health care delivery, of which only human beings can adequately provide for each human condition needing empathy, condolences, advice, salutation, compassion, companionship, and supervision.

Some of the technological medical devices available on the market today are the electronic health record, m-Health, portal technology, self-service kiosks, remote monitoring tools, sensors and wearables technology, real-time locating services, and pharmacogenomics/genome sequencing. Of all the listed medical technology devices available, we see the electronic health record, call light systems, and point of care devices to be the ones with widespread use in nursing homes demanding our attention as well. Each of these devices is not only noted for its own innovative and historical pathways, advantages, disadvantages, and areas of improvement, but also noted for not being a guarantee for a resident health outcome in and of itself.

The history of health records keeping, for example, has been long and tedious, deep into the efforts of many countries and professionals in the field of medicine, nursing, science, and technology. Most literature reviews have cited the Greeks, the Arabs, the Swedes, and the Egyptians as medical recordkeeping pioneers. They also saw the recordkeeping of births, deaths, and marriages of humans as being equally important throughout antiquity.

Specifically, the history of medical records is linked to the "doctors in history," dating back to the 1850s, naming Louis Pasteur, who introduced the germ theory and extended it to include investigation into the causes of many other diseases like TB and cholera. Other doctors in history of the same period who brought advancement in medicine included Joseph Lister and Edward Jenner, to name a few.

The father of medicine himself, Hippocrates, propounded the Hippocratic Oath for future physicians, and was also known to emphasize the principles of keeping all medical information confidential from everyone not involved in the treatment. By extrapolation, we now have the modern-day demand for health information privacy in accordance with the Health Insurance Portability and Accountability Act of 1996 (HIPAA) passed by the US Congress. The Hippocratic confidentiality of medical information and the "do no harm" in medical treatment principles enunciated to physicians, nurses, and indeed all health care practitioners, still stand today as a cornerstone in medical and nursing practice.

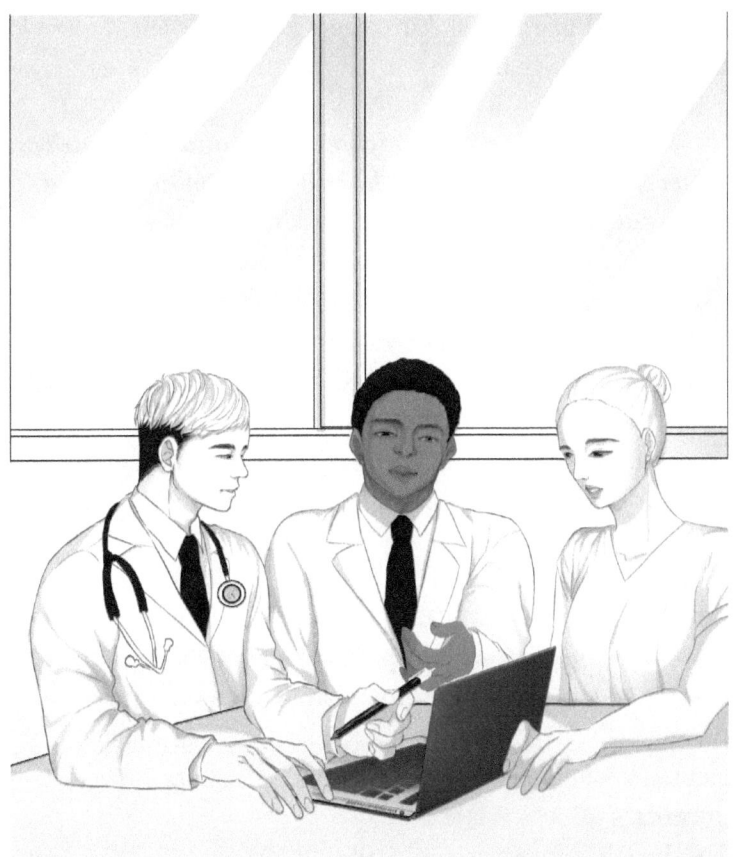

NURSING STAFF CARE-PLAN CONFERENCE
IN THE COMPUTER AGE

In ancient times, the proper method of recording and preserving medical information given the importance of confidentiality was problematic and obscure. Some of the methods frequently used in medical information recordkeeping ranged from memorization to written-down narratives. Gathering of medical information was conducted through observation and documenting patients' cures, complaints, and conversations about their medical issues. Accordingly, the first medical information gathering and written-down recordkeeping became attributed to the Greek astrologer-physicians Simon Forman and Richard Napier in the 1500s, who despite this pioneering achievement in medical recordkeeping and medical information gathering were nevertheless regarded as quark doctors. Wilkins (2011), in an article titled "How a Pair of Astrologers Helped Invent Modern Medical Record-Keeping," wrote that:

> *And yet, for all that, it's Forman and his equally disreputable protégé Richard Napier who have left a great gift to the history of medicine. The pair were astrologers, who took down detailed information about a patient's medical condition, then treated them through careful calculation of their astrological chart. While that might have not done much good for their patients, Forman and Napier's method had one huge benefit for posterity: they actually wrote down people's symptoms (Wikipedia, 2020, para 3).*

The modern Electronic Health Record (EHR) was introduced to the health care industry in 1920. Before then, it was the paper-based patient recordkeeping that was the predominant method, utilizing different styles of documenting health information, such as the problem-oriented medical record (POMR) and subjective, objective, assessment plan (SOAP) experimentations to assure efficiency in the recording and safekeeping of health records.

Even though the period of 1950–1970 is officially named the beginning of the Information Age, a.k.a. Computer Age, the paper and pencil documentation had continued into the 2000s for most industries, including healthcare. In health care in particular, medical information collected and documented on clipboards and notebooks led not only to medical errors and laborious work, but also the problem of keeping up with thicker medical record folders, requiring an additional staff training to "thin" them. Other problems associated with the traditional paper-based health information documentation were linked to poor penmanship and the accuracy of information recorded after time lapse between staff documentation and the event. Above all, handwritten medical record information was purely local to each medical establishment. But with the computerized clinical documentation, a warehouse in patient medical information is created for all end users.

Accordingly, in 2014, the Center for Medicare and Medicaid Services (CMS) mandated that health care facilities in the United States, through the Health Information Technology for Economic and Clinical Health (HITECH) Act of 2009, must implement electronic health records (EHR), a.k.a. EMR. Computerization of health information was also known as "going paperless."

Even though the electronic health record system is compatible with the spirit of holistic care management and has provided the possibility for different health care practitioners to vertically and horizontally gain access to health information on behalf of their comorbid patients, to move across different levels of care, there are worries about patient privacy and equipment malfunction. In general, modern health care technologies have been noted to improve patient care more in the medical perspective.

In nursing homes, a significant progress is noted when it comes to the storage, retrieval, and documentation of patient information. In short, health care practitioners are able to check in on their patients for decision-making, or collaborate with colleagues without having to physically visit the patient. The CMS interoperability rule mandating point of care (POC) documentation and the use of point click care (PCC) software devices was envisioned to allow health care information to be shared across organizational boundaries as an effective means of integrating, advancing, and improving healthcare services. PCC, which can be used remotely, was envisioned to help so that all care providers can have a better control of their organizational functions, monitor the progress of their patients, and have better access to communicate with other organizational members and subparts. The importance of POC-CNAs is significant because it is designed to capture and prevent the decline in residents' ADLs, which is the primary health reason most residents are admitted into nursing homes. To prevent a decline in residents' ADLs and apply appropriate and timely interventions, POC-CNA cannot be an off-site documentation. Rather, it is an on-site treatment and documentation of resident conditions defined as doing it, observing it, and documenting it, in that order.

Today, the use of computer and other clinical devices in both acute and LTC facilities for the periodic recording, reviewing, and updating of patient health status is not only widespread, it has resulted in an unprecedented reliance on the passive rather than active monitoring of patients by physicians and nurses. However, it is the point of care (POC) system, defined as an electronic bedside clinical documentation at the place and time of care, that is designed to bridge the gap between active and passive caregiving by allowing the caregiver to interact with patients while also documenting, making verbal transfer of health information from one practitioner to another a thing of the past. The best practice for caregivers is to read and act on others' computerized documentation as quickly and frequently as possible to avoid unutilized vital information. In situations where patients are sicker and dependent on others, there are some misgivings about how much staff reliance on the use of computer and other remote monitoring devices is affecting staff face-to-face direct patient supervision or their participation in care planning as required by OBRA '87.

In nursing homes, there is the belief that it is more of an active interpersonal relationship between staff and residents than the use of clinical devices that promotes resident quality of life and staff motivation. Patients who are bedridden and feeders, for example, would still require to be turned and repositioned, fed, and cleaned up by humans. Additionally, frequent rounding by nurses is beneficial as resident change in condition may require an immediate, on-the-spot intervention. It should not be forgotten that at the early stages of implementing electronic documentation and data collection many questions were put in perspective, questioning the value-added effects of computerized clinical documentation in nursing practice in general. In other words, can electronic devices do what humans can do to ultimately satisfy a patient's needs? In an article titled "Staff Experiences within the Implementation of Computer-Based Nursing Record in Residential Aged Care Facilities: a Systematic Review and Synthesis of Quantitative Research," MeiBner and Schnepp (2014) raised their skepticism about the advantages of electronic documentation, and posited that:

> *There is no empirical evidence that electronic nursing documentation systems add value to nursing, such as a) improved time management*

or b) improving information handling or c) increasing quality, the latter split in c1) quality of documentation (factual and professionally correct, continuous, complete) and c2) quality of care (more safety and better quality of life for the patients), (Wikipedia, 2020, para. 3).

Because in holistic nursing home management direct staff interaction with residents is seen as therapeutic, it is not only important to review how relevant the above statement is today as it was in 2014, but also to understand that by proxy staff are residents' families or relatives, who may no longer be available for their emotional support, or play the type of role that cannot be replaced by machines. Therefore, it becomes the function of the administrator to ensure appropriate balance between passive versus active care of residents within the concept of person-centered care, and that we do not abandon such humane activities that bind one human being to another to technology. There are some who would say that the usefulness of some medical technology in nursing homes is dependent on each resident's health condition and the activities of daily living (ADLs). In everyday life, modern technology has also given us the ability to email, text, or Tweet to our distant relatives, but these do not replace the intimacy of active visitation to our loved ones. In a health care setting, active care is operationally defined as the direct hands-on, face-to-face care and caring by health care providers, visitation, and family and community support systems as the resident's levels of functionality in ADLs declines.

Deciding how much of the medical technology to use versus the direct human intervention depends on the understanding of the meaning of resident-environment interaction needed to effectively care for the aging population, especially those residing in nursing homes.

In a nursing home setting, the quality of a resident's environment interaction constitutes the complementarity between the resident physical plant layout and the psychosocial and clinical needs of each resident to create wellness and ward off his/her feeling of isolation and loneliness. According to the "model of dynamic interaction" by Hooyman and Kiyak (1988.8–9), the concept of the "environmental press" further explains, emphasizing and defining the "demands that social and physical environments make on the individual to adapt, respond, or change." Adding, "the amount of press in an individual's living situation may range from minimal to quite high. For example, very little press is present in an institutional setting where an individual is not responsible for self-care."

OBRA '87's expectation requires institutions like nursing homes to have enough staff and resources to care for those who can no longer care for themselves. Accordingly, in an article titled "Appropriate Nurse Staffing Levels for U.S. Nursing Homes," Harrington et al. (2020) stated "on the whole, higher nurse staffing improves both the process and outcome measures of nursing home quality" (Wikipedia, 2020, para 2).

While there are merits to the demand to increase nurse staffing ratios, it should also be understood that quantity and quality in nursing home staffing are not always the same thing. In nursing homes, it is adequate staff training and effective supervision that produces quality staff unto nursing home quality. It should also be understood that nurse shortage, which has a negative impact on nursing home quality, is real but has not been sufficiently addressed. So far, the law of supply and demand has not corrected it. The regulatory mandate in and of itself is not enough. As a society, it is time to find new initiatives to grow the supply of nurses for nursing homes, especially among the "GNAs/CNAs" nursing assistants.

The goal of nursing home staffing in the holistic management perspective is to create a humanistic, homelike environment of care that is comprehensively conducive, not only to help residents to adjust to their current disabilities but also to monitor for future adjustments as may be necessary. To achieve wellness, it is important to assess the resident to determine his or her preference between active or passive care.

From a business perspective, and a note to the holistic nursing home manager, it is important that nursing home residents be seen and treated as customers with an option to choose another nursing home if the customer service in the current nursing home does not meet his/her expectation. When this concept of "customer" in nursing homes is perceived as it is perceived in other business enterprises, residents will seek improvement in the quality of service they receive with confidence.

This attitudinal change goes both ways. Employees must be trained not only to recognize the "power of choice" that residents and the families have, but also be transformed by it. When nursing home employees see residents as their customers as they see themselves as customers at Walmart or Macy's under the banner of the "customer bill of rights" in their heads, nursing home quality will improve because residents are able to exercise their power of self-determination and choice.

It should be noted that residents' admission into nursing homes is largely dependent on their ADLs and IADLs, ability to independently care for personal hygiene, incontinence management, dressing, feeding, and ambulating. The concept of instrumental activity of daily living (IADL), on the other hand, is asking the question relating to how much a person's lack of vital human senses, physical strength, and cognition can prevent him/her from independently cleaning and maintaining his house, managing money, moving around in the community, preparing meals, shopping for goods, taking his/her medication, dressing himself, and maintaining his/her personal hygiene. The level of diminishment in a person's ability in the above categories is what qualifies him/her for residency in different community facilities, including nursing homes. Today, however, through technological advancement in health, many elderly and infirm persons are able to live independently in the community longer than before.

Akin to the popularity and the widespread use of electronic health record (EHR) and computerized clinical documentation such as point of care (POC) in the health care community is call light technology. Like the EHR and the POC, call light has its advantages and disadvantages that the holistic nursing administrator must not ignore. The use of today's call light started from the concept of the servant's bell, whose name has changed from hand bell to call bell to nurse call, and dates back to the 1850s and the Crimean War. Florence Nightingale called it a hand bell and thought it was beneficial during the war to have this hand bell at each patient's bedside. Patients were required to ring the bell when they needed help. Today, healthcare facilities are required to ensure that call lights are available to all patients.

As part of environmental requirements in nursing homes, OBRA '87 F463.70 (F), under Resident Call System, states "the nurses' station must be equipped to receive resident call through a communication system from resident room, toilet and bathing facilities." The conditions for compliance are that the sound from the call light must be loud enough for staff to hear, that the mechanism of the call light must be within the residents' reach, must be functional, and must be responded to by staff in a timely manner.

Much as we have continued to view the call light positively within the patient-centered care concept, there are areas of noteworthiness that caregivers in nursing homes must bear in mind that call for a bridge between theory and practice about the importance of call lights. With all intents and purposes, call lights are designated to help in promoting resident safety, enhance residents' dignity, help staff prioritize their work, help staff in time management, and allow residents to have control in communicating with staff to have their needs met. Yet, the usefulness of call lights would depend on staff behavior and attitudes toward answering call lights timely, the ability of residents to reach and use call lights based on their physical disability or mental cognition, and the facility policy and practice on call lights.

Nursing home residents are required to be assessed on admission for ability to effectively use call lights as part of their demographic and orientation to the facility. This written documentation must be reviewed periodically to match the resident change in condition. As we stated earlier, one of the top complaints about nursing homes is the slow or lack of response to call light by staff when a resident needs help. When nursing home staff are not sufficiently trained as a matter of facility policy and resident assessment to empathize with the residents and their health condition, are not sufficiently aware of their residents' health condition associated with the call, or are desensitized by frequent call light calls, the tendency is for them to ignore the calls, to the detriment of the resident. A good nursing home policy on call lights should start by every staff being trained in role-play participation to recognize call light calls as a resident's emergency needing immediate response.

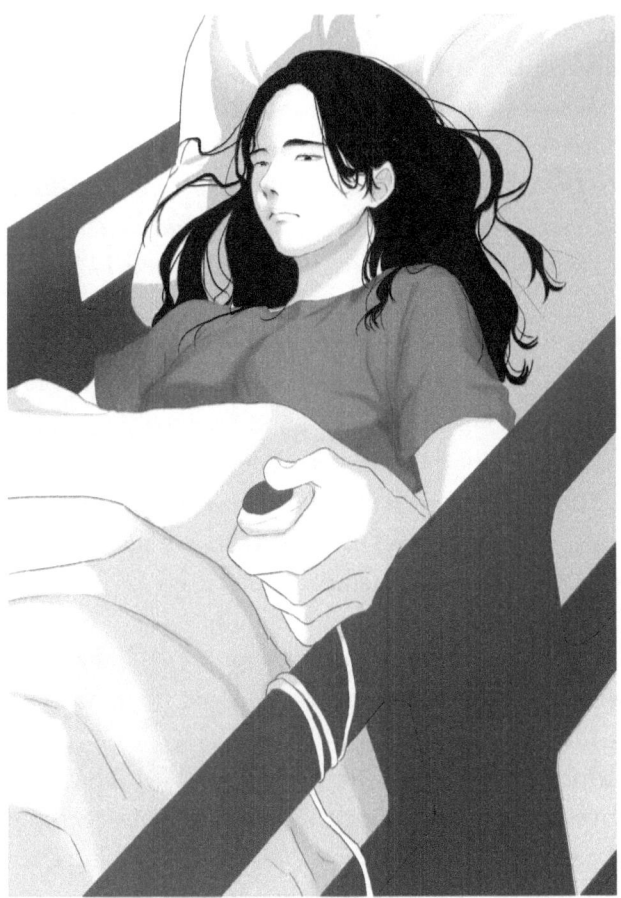

RESIDENT CARE AND NURSE CALL
SYSTEM IN NURSING HOMES

According to the research conducted by Galinato et al. (2016) titled "Perspective of Nurses and Patients on Call Lights Technology," it was found that staff were unclear on whose job it was to answer the call lights, with some staff members viewing call lights as an interruption to their workflow and delivery of patient care. Patients' comments

revealed issues of long wait times in getting their calls answered, inconsistencies with the response time, lack of follow through with requests and differing lengths of time to fulfill their requests . . .

call light response time to be a good predictor of key elements of patient satisfaction and that given the implication that nurses' responsiveness to call lights impact patient care quality and safety, changes in practice regarding call light use such as hourly rounding have been used to optimize call lights response times" (Wikipedia, 2019, para 1–2).

In a similar research paper titled "Perspectives of Patients and Families about the Nature of and Reasons for Call Light Use, and Staff Call Light Response Times," Tzeng (2011.225) found a compelling conclusion that "a patient who has used the call light and does not receive a timely response may attempt to do things independently (e.g. get out of bed to go to the bathroom) that might lead to a fall." The research also found families and visitors who participated in the study emphasized

the importance of answering of call light use in a timely manner because nurses' slow response to call light could result in toileting accidents and falls due to unattended attempts by patients to walk to the bathroom . . . participants perceived answering call light should be a priority among patient care tasks as a critical aspect of nursing staff roles

Either in the community or in health care institutions, the use of clinical technology and devices is gaining strength and credited for saving or prolonging lives. As the population from the greatest generation, the silent and the baby boomer generations is increasing, older, and sicker, they will require hands-on, face-to-face assistance from caregivers to fulfil the philosophical mandates associated with holistic care. The assumption is that it will happen amidst the decreasing number of caregivers and stay-home family members. Also, due to the impending shortage of nurses, such as in nursing homes and other health care institutions, the increase in telehealth and telemedicine will be required to supplement human labor, but not replace it.

Chapter 12

Leadership and Holistic
Management in Nursing Homes

So far, we have documented related theories, assumptions, and benefits stemming from the holistic approach to managing organizations, especially nursing homes. But for any organization, old or new, to function, it must operate under the right kind of leadership to ensure its holistic growth and development; moreover, its survival.

In general, organizational leaders are often characterized and evaluated based on their leadership qualities, traits, and leadership styles affecting the performance of their organizations. Key theorists frequently associated with theorizing and analyzing leadership qualities, traits, and styles for future leaders to explore are Kurt Lewin for authoritarian, participative, and delegative leadership; Bernard M. Bass for transformational leadership; Max Weber for transactional leadership; and Hersey and Blanchard for situational leadership. Today, it is the longstanding demand for improvement in nursing home quality that tends to put the industry's leadership at a crossroad of change in management approach and continuous public outcry and dissatisfaction with its operation.

In an article titled "Nursing Home Safety: Current Issues and Barriers to Improvement," Gruneir and Mor (2008) wrote, "the past few decades have seen increasing concerns about the quality of nursing home (NH) care. As with other health care sectors, NHs have attempted to embrace a culture of safety, but the additional barriers that they face place the NH industry at a distinct disadvantage" (Wikipedia, 2020, para 1).

Business competition is a reality of life, and the nursing home industry is no exception. In the last century or so, the business practice of "if it isn't broken, don't fix it" was acceptable. Not anymore. In today's market economies, businesses like nursing homes must compete well and respond to the demand of the consumers in order to survive well, as opposed to just limping along.

Beating business competition is not a new concept, but one that is an important adjunct to management functions, requiring the type of leadership that is future-looking to anticipate, experiment, and imagine change. It is this assumption that fits the narrative of Thomas Friedman, quoted as "what every employer is looking for is not someone who can do the job, but someone who can re-invent the job." Also, from the framework of holistic management perspective, there is increased requirement for leaders to be able to satisfactorily "balance internal needs and to adapt to environmental circumstances" (Wikipedia, 2020, para.2)

This chapter is not intended to relegate much of the existing management theories on the subject of leadership. Rather, it is intended to help steer current and future leaders in the direction of embracing how to achieve better management outcomes by exploring areas of organizational leadership critical to holistic management: the definition and function of a leader/manager in an organization, whether leaders are born or made, locus of leadership in organization, importance of leadership traits, qualities, temperament, and leadership style, especially in holistic management. Consequently, there exists a need to discuss that leaders thrive when they do not only embrace change but also understand the implications and use of power and authority; and by reviewing related leadership concepts and leadership styles, they can properly reevaluate their on-the-job leadership performance in light of their organizational goal and the cliché that aptly applies to leaders of organizations "to whom much is given, much is expected"—or should we say, "uneasy lies the head that wears a crown."

In an article titled "Leadership Styles in Relation to Employees' Trust and Organizational Change Capacity: Evidence from Non-profit Organizations," Yasir, Imran, Irshad, Mohamad, and Khan (2016) emphasized the importance of leadership and leadership styles in organizations, and wrote: "the importance of leadership has grown significantly in organizations as compared with the past . . . business environment is changing and becoming impulsive and volatile" (Wikipedia 2020, para 1). To them, a leader's trustworthiness and managing change were directly linked to a successful leadership style. In much the same vein, Bethel (1990, 123), in a book titled "Making a Difference: 12 Qualities that Make You a Leader," wrote: "leadership style isn't what you think your style is: It's what others perceive it to be. Like beauty, leadership is in the eye of the beholder."

From time immemorial, behavioral theorists of organizational development (OD) and management development (MD) persuasions have provided answers to the above organizational topics, mostly reflecting different situational factors and perspectives on organizational leadership. In OD, it is implied that leaders who want to be successful must concern themselves with the workings of organizational structure, activities, resources, programs, theories, processes, communication, and change patterns, staff assignment, and morale, etc., as well as MD, which denotes the extent to which leaders and staff are utilizing educational means to improve their skills to meet organizational goals. These theoretical foundations are profound in today's management practice and how leaders should lead/manage modern organizations.

Postulating that all leadership/management requirements are not the same for all organizations and that organizations differ in terms of their purpose, structure, and goals is in support of transition toward the holistic management approach in personal, business, and health care management. Therefore, the existing variation in definitions, assumptions, and theories in much of these behavioral science literatures relating to who a leader is, his leadership function, leadership style, and supervisory management are available in recognition of the changing nature of organizations to provoke continuous formal and informal education and the curiosity of the practicing leaders and managers to learn, emulate, and perfect their trades in relationship to holistic management.

Managing a nursing home to achieve nursing home quality requires a full understanding of its characteristics in order to apply appropriate management style and supervision. Nursing homes, for the most part, are staffed with direct care nurses, administration and support staff with varying degrees of management and supervisory skills and expertise that may not be sufficient to increase or maintain nursing home quality. A study conducted by Poel et al. (2020) titled "Leadership Styles and Leadership Outcomes in Nursing Homes: A Cross-Sectional Analysis" found leadership styles in nursing homes not transformational but passive-avoidant, and wrote "results indicate that passive-avoidant leadership styles are excessively present in contrast to transformational leadership styles in nursing homes. This highlights an urgent need to invest in leadership development" (Wikipedia 2020, para, 5). Passive-avoidant leadership style describes a manager who pays little or no attention to employees' behavior until something goes wrong.

Understanding Leadership Styles and Holistic Management

In the main, the importance of leadership, either in the traditional management or holistic management approach, is to influence and inspire others to meet organizational goals as implicated in leadership styles. Succinctly, when Holland (2017) wrote his article titled "What Is Leadership and Why Does it Matter to Me," he was raising an important question of self-awareness to practitioners in relation with their leadership style, stating "your leadership style is a melting pot of your personality, your life experiences, your natural/preferred communication style, the level of your emotional intelligence, and your perspective" (Wikipedia, 2020, para. 2). If so, what is the big deal about holistic leadership, and why does it require a different leadership style from the traditional leadership?

The benefits of holistic management that are not deployed by the traditional management approach have already been given to include the behavioral characteristic of leadership and the motivational aspects of all of the organizational members. Consequently, in an article titled "9 Characteristics of Holistic Leaders," Funk (2016) emphasized and wrote:

> *Traditional leadership competence has been about behavior—what a leader is capable of doing in the workplace. That approach describes desired*

actions but it overlooks the character traits that are crucial for guiding those actions. A more complete model of leadership competence goes beyond actions to describe who the leader is as a person. I refer to this model as holistic leadership. Holistic leaders know how to integrate their character and values into their leadership, and they understand that they bring their whole selves to their leadership role— body, mind and spirit (Wikipedia, 2020, para 1).

In another article, titled "Holistic Leadership," Larcher (2011) clarified the difference between traditional leadership and holistic leadership, and wrote:

Holistic leadership is an approach to leadership that incorporates not only WHAT leaders need to do and HOW they need to do it, but also the WHO and WHERE of leadership. It's not just about acquiring some leadership skills or techniques or behaviours, it's about aligning the whole person-intellect, emotions, spirituality and behaviours (Wikipedia 2020, para 1).

It is worthy of note that most organizations, including nursing homes, today are large-scale and decentralized, requiring that we examine the impact of change on today's organizational leadership. Unlike in the days of sole-proprietorships and partnerships in business operations, today's corporate organizational charts are showing myriad functional leaders in different physical operational locations thousands of miles apart. Given the scenario that all organizational members, especially the leadership team, must stay connected, we are reminded to review what constitutes an approach to holistic management.

The block-by-block structure in the corporate management process is designed so that each leader, by becoming the areal person in charge of his block, ensures that he not only achieves his essential management functions but also stays connected within the entire corporate system.

Whenever the naming interorganizational leaders by functional areas is necessitated, systems of assuring an individual or collective productivity, responsibility, and accountability are also necessitated. As indicated earlier, corporatization of nursing homes makes managing nursing homes of today an example where departmentalization, decentralization, and assignment of departmental or divisional leaders are occurring and cannot be avoided. Henri Fayol (1841–1925) theorized that each leader be responsible for carrying out his basic management functions of "forecasting, planning, organizing, commanding, coordinating and controlling," a.k.a. "Fayol's six primary functions of management" (Wikipedia, 2020, para 1) in addition to "Fayol's 14 principles of management."

It is noteworthy that we are using the terms *manager* and *leader* interchangeably without ignoring the subtle difference in meaning between them. Unlike most contemporary authors, early management/organizational theorists like Rensis Likert were consistent in the use of management as in "management style," instead of "leadership style." So what would the error be if someone is to ask you what your management style or leadership style is? Very little. However, Northouse (2013, 12–13), in a book titled "Leadership: Theory and Practice," has shed some light, stating that "leadership is a process that is similar to management in many ways. Leadership involves influence, as does management . . . to manage means to accomplish activities and master routines, whereas to lead means to influence others and create visions for change."

Concerning the frequently asked questions about a leader being born or made, or what makes a good or bad leader, we are reminded once again of being in the intersection of human trait and the environmental (in-born or learned) factors as determinants of human behavior. It often boils down to nature versus nurture in deciphering what determines a good leader and a bad one. Northouse's definition of leadership as "a process whereby an individual influences a group of individuals to a common goal" (p.5) clarifies that leadership "is not a trait or characteristic that resides in a leader, but rather a transactional event that occurs between the leader and the followers" (p.5).

When we refer to in-born, natural, or innate leadership qualities, we mean those qualities that may relate aggressiveness, assertiveness; empathy, charisma; self-confidence and social abilities; and communication/oration, oftentimes associated with the so-called natural born leaders. While we do not dispute that these are some leadership qualities that can come naturally in some people, we also support other existing theories that leadership qualities are not only skills that can come from formal training and experience but that which requires a lifetime activity to acquire new skills relative to changes in an organization.

When we stated earlier that all organizations as well as their leadership requirements are not the same, we were alluding to the reality of leaders who can be successful in one leadership situation but completely fail in another. To squelch the ongoing nature versus nurture or chicken and egg controversy in leadership, Riggio (2020), in an article titled "Leaders: Born or Made," stated that "the best estimates offered by research is that leadership is about one-third born and two-thirds made" (Wikipedia, 2020, para 1). Consequently, we see the continuous efficacy and likelihood of leadership development training that will include holistic management to increase, not decrease in higher education, workshops, in services, and practice.

In an article titled "Leadership Development and Leadership Effectiveness," Amagoh (2020) agreed and wrote "it is important that organizations embark on leadership development programs that will enhance leadership effectiveness" (Wikipedia, 2020, para 1). In a book titled "Management of Organizational Behavior: Leading Human Resources," Hersey, Blanchard and Johnson (2001, 11) explained further and wrote:

> Whether leadership can be learned is an issue that has perplexed researchers for decades and one that has important implications for readers of this book. If leaders are born, why spend time reading and developing your skills . . . if leaders are made, then everyone can become a leader, and there is hope for us all

The late Martin Luther King Jr. (1929–1968), who is always remembered as an excellent leader during the civil rights movement in the United States, is known to have possessed most of the leadership qualities we have listed above. As someone who can be called a born leader, most of his nonviolent skills and techniques to protest racism and discrimination in the United States were admittedly learned from the teachings of Mahatma Gandi (1869–1948), who himself used nonviolent means to fight and defeat British rule in India. Accordingly, the former president of the United States, John F. Kennedy (1917–1963) stated that "leadership and learning are indispensable."

In a nursing home setting, the licensed administrator is its leader, whose leadership style is required to accommodate the nature of nursing home operation. In nursing home management, there exist several different areas of clinical/technical operations where separate miniature leaders are required. These are leaders in this organization who make technical/clinical decisions toward meeting the organizational goal and vision. The roadmap to a successful management lies in the administrator's ability as the leader to embark on establishing a clear vision and oversight for the organization, which includes managing decentralization in leadership functions, establishing report and communication links, motivating employees, guiding and supporting subordinates in their work performance, and building subordinates' morale. As we discussed earlier, we must also keep in mind that the licensed administrator is responsible and held accountable for all decisions made on his behalf. As the person in charge of the day-to-day operation, understanding subordinates' skill levels and their leadership role is critical to enhance their training and motivation and communication.

In practice, the administrator's limitation in authority may occur depending on the supervisory attitudes and behavior of corporate officers and the organizational structure. By understanding and embracing the benefits accruing from participative management as an arm of a holistic management approach, it is important for nursing home administrators to decry disunity from any part of their organization. To this end, it is critical that interviewers selecting leaders for organizations for nursing homes consider candidates' leadership traits, qualities, temperament, style, as well as his technical/clinical skills, among other things, to ensure a match relating to the purpose, goal, and objectives of the organization.

For an example, in nursing homes, there are departmental leaders with staff, budgetary, and supervisory responsibilities, even though the overall responsibility and accountability of ensuring regulatory compliance and profitability of the business rest on the licensed administrator. As such, his leadership style requires that he is multi-tasked, flexible, and knowledgeable.

By reporting directly to government agencies, his corporate office, managing staff behavior, managing change, and assuring organizational outcomes, it is fair to say that the licensed administrator's leadership ability is always on the line. The good-fit assumption, particularly in nursing homes, is based on the necessity to avoid a mismatch in leadership abilities that are suited for the industry, department, or group. For example, the leadership skills needed in the construction industry would not be suitable in the health care industry, and vice versa. Accordingly, hiring managers are often tasked to determine the goodness of fit since not all potential leaders may be sufficiently eclectic to be able to adjust their leadership styles and behavior in response to diverse situational changes the organization demands, brought about by such factors as technology, sociocultural changes, education, regulations, and clientele. Being an eclectic leader assures personal preference, freedom, and self-sufficiency, knowing that a leadership style is not prescriptive but self-selective from an array of styles a leader has already learned. His preference depends on which leadership style he believes to be more applicable to the organizational situation at hand.

Some of the leadership styles that are contained in much of the business management literatures for your review and continuous reading are democratic, autocratic, laissez-faire, strategic, transformative, transactional, coach style, bureaucratic, and participative. For beginners in leadership positions, the frequently asked question needing an address is which of the leadership style works best. According to research, the truth is there is no one-size-fits-all. It all depends; meaning, you decide which leadership style fits your unique situation. As suggested in Hersey-Blanchard's situational leadership theory, written by Cherry (2019), "no single leadership style is best. Instead, it depends on which type of leadership and strategies are best-suited to the task" (Wikipedia, 2020, para 1).

In a situational leadership theory, the leadership style used is based on the maturity of each group, rotating from telling, selling, participating, and delegating. While most organizational goals are monolithic, the process of meeting them requires the application of the management functions mentioned above to understand the organizational characteristics and to determine the needs of each intergroup of the organization. In most organizations like nursing homes, whereby different groups of employees with different skill sets are required to perform different functions to holistically meet the organizational goal, it is important to comply with the Hersey-Blanchard situational leadership theory and the definition of an organization as:

> a social unit of people that is structured and managed to meet a need or to pursue collective goals. All organizations have a management structure that determines relationships between the different activities and the members and subdivides and assigned roles, responsibilities, and authority to carry out different tasks . . . the leadership functions to plan, organize, lead, and control is implicated in the definition that organization is the structural framework of duties and responsibilities required of personnel in performing various functions with a view to achieve business goals through organization (Wikipedia 2020, para 1).

Also noted is Rensis Likert, who advocated participative management style in his management systems approach, implying the importance of cultural inclusiveness and systems integration as the backbone of a workforce that is holistic. Consequently, both Rensis Likert and Hersey-Blanchard's pathways to leadership have become aptly applicable to nursing home holistic management only when leaders are able to advocate, promote, and combine workforce cultural inclusiveness, systems integration initiatives with group-specific or individualized staff development programs, and adapt to situational changes in their organizations.

In much the same vein, Fred E. Fieldler (1922–2017), in his contingency theory, saw organizations as "open systems," and management effectiveness as depending on the leader's ability to manage organizational variabilities through an ability to apply different leadership styles in different situations. Consequently, contingency theory is defined as:

An organizational theory that claims that there is no best way to organize a corporation, to lead a company, or to make decisions. Instead, the optimal course of action is contingent (dependent) upon the internal and external situation. A contingent leader effectively applies their own style of leadership to the right situation. Contingent leaders are flexible in choosing and adapting to succinct strategies to suit change in situation at a particular period in time in the running of the organization (Wikipedia, 2020, para 1).

Understanding the Concept of Power and Authority within Holistic Management

Leadership is often regarded as the engine of an organization, with the responsibility to holistically connect all the dots from a wide variety of internal and external situations, and manage employee behavior transitioning from home life to work life. Akin to leadership is the concept of power and authority, as in personal power and positional power, usually expressed also as informal and formal power respectively. Power and authority can be defined as vital ingredients of leadership that help the leader to get things done.

Organizational leadership in holistic management is about establishing, first all, the relevant parts there are in an organization and how they are connected in order to be able to make effective decisions for change as necessary. Second, leadership is about using the tools of management to understand and manage employee behavior. In all of the industrialized societies, a person's home life and work life have been found not to be mutually exclusive.

Consequently, all societies are expected to produce able-bodied, well-bred, well-behaved, and well-skilled citizenry in order for them to be productive and prosperous. Research studies have shown how childhood upbringing relates to a positive or negative adulthood behavior, and how external events can affect the internal operational efficiency of an organization. In a 1989 fact-based movie titled *Lean on Me*, it is shown that when one of the students, Kaneesha Carter, developed maladjusted behavior while in high school, the school principal, Joe Clark, was able to trace this problem to the student's home environment. Omere (2017), in an article titled "7 Ways Parents Work to Destroy Their Child's Future Success," posited "the effect of bad parenting on the children include antisocial behavior, poor resilience, depression, and aggression . . . as they grow into adults" (Wikipedia, 2020, para.2 and 9).

While it is not uncommon to use the concepts of power and authority interchangeably, Surbhi (2016) shed more light and wrote:

> When the question is about influencing or manipulating others, two things that go side by side in the field of management are power and authority . . . many of us think that these two terms are one and the same thing, but there exists a fine line of difference between power and authority. While the former is exercised in a personal capacity, the latter is used in a professional capacity (Wikipedia 2020, para 1).

Conjointly, power and authority reflect someone's ability and knowledge in organization to both govern and make effective decisions affecting the actions of others relative to political, technical, clinical, financial, or personal issues. The leader's ability to effectively govern and make decisions is further explained within the context of how power and authority, formal and informal, are used, as well as how they are perceived by others.

Further distinction between a formal and informal authority in leadership is that a formal authority is based on one's organizational title or rank, while informal authority is based on one's related work skills—clinical, technical, or interpersonal. In a technically/clinically oriented work environment like nursing homes, it is not uncommon for the holder of position of power or formal authority in organization to see himself as omnipotent, even though it is the holder of personal power or informal authority who is the gatekeeper to the company's continuous existence based on know-how and productivity.

In an article titled "Uncovering 2 Types of Authority," Grensing-Pophal (2019) pointed out that "in contrast to the formal leader, the informal leader is someone who does not have the official authority to direct the group. Despite this, the group chooses to follow the lead of this person" (Wikipedia, 2020, para 2). The legacy of classical management is the arrangement by hierarchical formal ranks and titles. While there should be no quarrel with internal set-up of organizations, it is worthwhile to keep in mind that in holistic management, what matters the most is the leader's holistic view—an opportunity one has to ensure that, organizationally, all parts is not only the whole, but something greater than the whole.

To assure the efficacy of leadership, either in classical or holistic management, it is important for a leader to explore and fully understand not only the concepts of power and authority in an organization but also the implications of a leader's deficiency in not possessing both. Personal power, which is linked to expert power, is defined as all the prerequisites of skills a leader must possess above and beyond that of his subordinates. In this regard, personal/expert power is not what the leader perceives of himself; rather, it is the perception that subordinates have about their leader's knowledge base, which they believe is sufficient enough to supplement that which they do not have.

It is in this regard that Jim Rohn (1930–2009) is quoted as saying, "a good objective of leadership is to help those who are doing poorly to do well and those who are doing well to do even better." And John Quincy Adams (1767–1848), former president of the United States of America, is quoted as saying, "if your actions inspire others to dream more, learn more, do more and become more, you are a leader."

In a book titled *The One Minute Manager*, Blanchard and Johnson (1982, 10) wrote that "the people who work with you as their manager will look to you as one of their sources of wisdom." On the other hand, position of power is defined as the control a leader wields over the machinery of his organization and the behavior of others using his formal authority. Again, we are faced with the chicken and egg scenario. Can we have a chicken without the egg, and vice versa? Or put another way, can a child without two parents providing parental guidance or raised by a single parent grow up to be a productive citizen? This is a moral question and remains virtually an open question. However when leadership in organizations is expressed as a means of providing "support systems," it confirms the old adage that "two heads are better than one."

Leading a formal or an informal organization is more than gathering a bunch of people and equipment under one roof. Leaders under the holistic management approach must learn the art of treating their subordinates as "family." Philosophically, the beginning of a human organization is the biological human family. Business organizations comprising a formal leader and employees can be likened to a biological human family, comprising parents, children, and some extended family; not only because they both need structure, rules, codes of conduct, and leadership, but also that most behaviors (good or bad) exhibited in formal organizations may owe their origins from their biological human family, and vice versa.

As far-fetched as this comparison may look to some people, it has a far-reaching implication to the society as a whole. Furthermore, it is not unheard of for a formal business leader to refer to his subordinates as his "extended family," if not for anything else but to demonstrate endearment toward cooperation. Not uncommon either to hear a leader of a formal organization asking his subordinates to "keep any bad behavior at home," or a parent who hears his working child using profane language at home questioning him where he learned it from.

Ideally, for our society to function optimally, the perception is that both formal organizations and biological families need to play a role of becoming promulgators of moral values and work ethics. In an article titled "A Home from Home: the Organization as Family" (Brown and McCartney, 2007) wrote:

> *The basic unit of human organization has always been the family . . . we provide analogies between the notions of "family" as a private social institution and the work organization, drawing no conclusions, but providing some small insights into affinities and congruence which blur the private/public distinction. If we assert anything at all, it is this: because the work organization is family, we are able to slip from one to the other each day with the minimum of psychic stress (Wikipedia, 2020 para 1–2).*

In this scenario, it is by design that someone with authority—usually the father and mother, an elderly person in the family, or a formal leader in an organization—becomes responsible for the nurturing, problem-solving, structural arrangement, and disciplinary action needs that may arise within the organization. While a biological human family is often referred to as an informal organization, the similarity existing between the biological human family and a formal business organization is that they both involve human relationships, requiring the exercise of moral values, leadership, authority, and the desire for all to survive well.

Accordingly, the prerequisite for managing either a biological human family or a formal organization lies in the leader's emotional intelligence— tendencies relating to compassion, empathy, self-awareness, setting good examples, self-control, patience, ethics, and ability to understand the emotion of others. Parents who raise children at home need these qualities as well as leaders of people in the workplace. A parent is the head of the household, and the head of a formal organization is the formal leader.

In both analogies, the exercise of personal power and positional power is inherently important to achieve the same goal of shaping or managing group behavior. Even though personal power and positional power tend to be implicitly expressed within the biological family but explicitly expressed within a formal organization, the desired goal is the same in directing another human being to "do the right thing."

There is a holistic virtuous circle connection between the biological family upbringing of an individual, his schooling, and his workforce participation. By nature, modern societies cannot survive without following this key part of the human development process. Our societies are designed to produce skilled labor to produce and deliver goods and services. In this scenario, it is an African proverb that explains it all: "it takes a village to raise a child." Motivating, nurturing, and redirecting the activities of another individual to be a productive member of society has become a function of the family, educators, and workplace leadership, realizing that in our world of work, a productive workforce that leads to a good life in society is achieved with good and productive people. While the family upbringing of a child lays the foundation for the child to succeed in later years, his formal schooling and workforce participation are helpful in defining his standing in society.

Leaders of these institutions must be mindful of their impact on the societal well-being as a whole. The most frequently asked question is, can a leader successfully lead any organization without the security of both personal and positional powers? To most behavioral science experts, the answer would be clearly no. Positional power in the absence of personal or expert power leads to an eventual loss of the leader's reverence from subordinates, and may instead inherit an additional title from them of "empty suit." Comparatively, the loss of respect from children could only come because their parents have lost or abused their personal or positional power. It is not enough for parents to use the "I brought you into this world and I can take you out" approach, or a formal leader to use a "shape up or ship out" approach in staff behavioral management. It is important to note that both domains of power are technically essential requirements in leadership if an organization is to function, but it is personal power that is deemed more likely to inspire and influence others to do well.

Personal power is the leader's internalized powerhouse, which subordinates rely on for problem-solving needs, while positional power is the shell from where his external strength to govern is executed. Because today's organizations are people oriented, with different technical/clinical skills, they need management through collaboration, cooperation, and participation, rather than that of command and control. When formal organizational leaders meaningfully exhibit both positional and personal powers, they are seen in the eyes of their subordinates as legitimate and referent. The same interpretation applies to parents, who do not receive enough credit for their contribution to raising the workforce of the future. For leaders who embark on holistic management, we therefore recommend that they view all objects from the perspective of PPF—past, present, and future, remembering the old adage that "a fruit does not fall far from the tree."

Chapter 13

Understanding Employees' Motivation in the Holistic Management Perspective

Staff motivational program is a work-life need satisfaction program that organizations use to satisfy the social needs, emotional needs, and financial needs of their employees. As complicated as implementing an effective staff motivational program may seem to be, it is essential for all organizations if the machinery of management is to operate smoothly and consistently. Management's investment in a staff motivational and reinforcement program is directly correlated with staff productivity when they are adequately calibrated.

Motivation is defined as a process of an individual's need to initiate and maintain his goal-oriented activities, while reinforcement is the reward for an individual to strengthen/encourage his future behavior/achievement. There is an idiomatic expression of "putting the cart before the horse," meaning doing something in the wrong order. The reality is, it is the horse that is capable of pulling the cart, and by reversing the order and emphasizing the cart rather than the horse, the desirable organizational goal can be unachievable. In this scenario, we liken the horse to employees who require motivation and the cart being the desire of management to achieve a certain production level. Unfortunately, with respect to the relationship between staff motivation, reinforcement, and staff work performance, there are still managers who tend to put more emphasis first on staff performance without due consideration to what causes staff performance to improve. Employees who have positive feeling about themselves, their jobs, and accorded with positive reinforcement will be productive.

There are two basic parts to staff motivation that is noteworthy—intrinsic and extrinsic motivation. Intrinsic motivation is the extent to which an employee likes the job itself without regard for any external reward. Extrinsic motivation is the extent to which an employee's external reward (salaries, recognition, fame, cash bonuses, and gifts) matches his expectation for doing a job.

One of the frequently asked questions is whether intrinsic motivation is more important than extrinsic motivation, and vice versa. Proponents of intrinsic motivation believe it provides a sustainable staff performance while extrinsic motivation provides an intermittent staff performance. While there are many opinions and diverse answers to this important question, we see the efficacy of staff motivation as lying in the healthy interaction of intrinsic motivation, extrinsic motivation, and the sustainability of the motivational plan itself. However, in nursing homes, the administrator must decide which motivation program is more likely to bring change in parts of the organization where problems exist—monetary reward or work itself.

Some answers to this argument have been presented in the two-factor theory of Frederick Herzberg. And in much of the industrial psychology research, the finding is that there is a direct correlation between employees' motivation levels, their well-being on the job, and productivity. Accordingly, Quain (2019), in an article titled "Positive & Negative Effects of Employee Motivation," wrote:

> To run a successful business, your employees must feel valued. One of the most effective ways of accomplishing this goal is motivating employees through various types of incentives. In some cases, incentives might be monetary such as bonuses or gifts for exceeding performance standards . . . however it's important that you understand the pros and cons of employee motivational techniques so that you can avoid setting the wrong precedent (Wikipedia, 2020, para. 1–2).

Suffice to say that since Hawthorne experiment, the art of keeping staff motivated as a function of productivity has become one of the most challenging parts of management. As Blanchard and Johnson (1982 13) noted, the challenge for change is likely to be more on some of today's managers, who still describe themselves as "tough managers whose organizations seemed to win while their people lost . . . autocratic manager keeps on top of the situation, a bottom-line manager, hard-nosed, realistic, profit minded."

Based on the Hawthorne experiment by Elton Mayo (1880–1949), the new era of the neoclassical management theory was born to advocate for a focus on the human side of an organization and the social needs of employees as a precursor for cultural change in organizations, for a win-win situation for both the organization and employees, defining a new type of relationship between management and employees. While neoclassical management did not seek to replace the concept of standardization posed by classical management, it did bring the man versus machine controversy to a close. Henceforth, man would no longer be treated as an adjunct to a machine, but separately, as an individual with basic human needs, including emotional needs, that must be satisfied; and for management to learn the proverb that "you can catch more flies with honey than with vinegar."

In most human resources literature, staff motivational programs have been referred to as either staff engagement, staff incentive, or staff motivation programs. Because each program is titled differently. They are likely to carry different meanings, limitations, and interpretations. The less comprehensive and more fragmented these programs are, the less likely for them to succeed.

Given the fact that there is no simple or one correct answer to what motivates employees to be more productive, organizations will stand to benefit from a consolidated title of "staff motivational engagement and incentive program," which is comprehensive and holistic. The concept of motivational engagement and incentive program is coined and introduced herein to provide human resources managers a fuller understanding of what it takes to enhance employees' job satisfaction and productivity.

In an article titled "73 Employee Engagement Ideas for Any Budget," Madlingler (2019) wrote: "even the best tools and technology can't keep your business going when your people are unhappy and unmotivated" (Wikipedia, 2020, para.1). She went on to present seventy-three nonmonetary motivational ideas worthy of our recommendation for organizations to consider when planning their employee needs satisfaction program. Madlinger's ideas further confirm that for an organization to thrive, its leadership must have a well-developed, effective, and well-resourced staff motivational engagement and incentive program beyond temporary and misguided cash bonuses. Even though in today's economy money is very important, it does not encompass all aspects of human needs.

In an article titled "Why the Millions We Spend on Employee Engagement Buy Us So Little," Morgan (2017) warned against short-sighted employee needs satisfaction plans, and wrote:

> *Organizations are spending hundreds of millions of dollars on employee engagement programs, yet their scores on engagement surveys remain abysmally low. How is that possible? Because most initiatives amount to an adrenaline shot. A perk is introduced to boost scores, but over time the effect wears off and scores go back down . . . when organizations make real gains, it's because they're thinking long-term (Wikipedia, 2020, para. 1).*

According to research studies, most organizations have an estimated payroll budget of 1 percent to 10 percent for staff motivational engagement and incentive programs. Similar studies have also found such an investment to have a positive and direct relationship with staff job performance, morale, cooperation, and commitment. But the caution that exists is that the direct relationship of staff motivation and productivity cannot only be measured by how much more productive employees are but also by their willingness to perform.

The concept of "willingness to perform" and "employee happiness" is echoed by industrial psychologists as an important part of staff motivation. It implies that both the manager and the employee perceive that someone is doing his job enthusiastically. Creating a motivated workplace is a part of organizational development and organizational management, in which the staff motivational engagement and incentive program must be comprehensive, sustainable, continuous, and inclusive. To be "comprehensive" means considering the complex nature of human beings and the totality of their needs; "sustainable" means a staff motivational practice that is a long-term project; "continuous" means implementing staff needs satisfaction strategy as a steady stream toward employees' needs fulfilment, uninterrupted by the whims and caprices of the employer; and "inclusive" means fairness and equal treatment for all.

The payoff in creating a motivated workplace is beneficial to an organization, resulting in higher productivity, retention rates, and company loyalty, as well as good customer relationships among staff. In a holistic management, staff willingness toward participation, cooperation, and collaboration is inherent not only in their willingness to learn new methods of production or rendering services, but also in their willingness to contribute more for the common good. In the same token, it is by embracing staff motivation that holistic management is regarded as being more capable of managing ethno-cultural diversity and workforce inclusiveness for all organizational stakeholders than does the traditional management.

The holistic organizational philosophy of "not leaving any organizational stone unturned" or "not leaving any organizational member behind" is therefore seen as consistent with the need for organizations to establish a formal process for nurturing their staff through the understanding of staff motivation. Organizations must identify and separate individual needs from group needs, with the understanding that as a matter of practice there is no one magic bullet or a one-size-fits-all plan. All fingers are not the same. One employee may have a financial need while another may have the need for a change in workload, and so on. For too many managers who must decide which motivational button to push for optimum result, this is where the rubber meets the road, and the time for managers to reach deep into their knowledge base and personal experience.

Realizing how competitive today's workforce has become with staff shortages, buying and selling of goods and services and so forth, budgeting enough money, time, and effort in designing and implementing staff motivation cannot be overemphasized. In an article titled "Budgeting for Employee Engagement," (Bailey 2018) observed that the millennial workers "who represent a significant portion of the workforce, expect more from their workplace than just a salary and benefits" (Wikipedia, 2020, para.1). It is to this end that staff motivation cannot be random but targeted toward staff individual or group needs, with assurance of cause and effect relationship. It is also worthwhile to remember that a staff motivation program that is not implemented fairly can do more harm than good.

According to literature reviews, there are as many benefits as there are side effects to staff motivation that all leaders of organizations must be aware of, especially those who practice holistic management with the goal of keeping all parts of the organization integrated, functional, and productive. The following points must be borne in mind. A motivational program that is poorly designed and implemented can cause workplace conflicts and engender selfishness. For example, it may cause employees to focus narrowly only on the goal that they believe will bring them more rewards, causing them to stop producing upon reaching the predetermined goal. Some employees who feel that the process of incentive distribution is discriminatory, unfair, and tilted to favor certain employees may exhibit negative attitudes toward the company and those employees. It is also noteworthy that a staff motivation and incentive program can be regarded as meaningless if it is not implemented to build a lasting relationship and goodwill between employees and the organization and prevent organizational problems, and instead deployed short-term, usually in the form of cash bonuses after problems have already erupted. We cannot emphasize enough that a staff motivational engagement and incentive program works best when it is designed not only as a long-term maintenance plan, but as part of the initial organizational design and development, with room for improvement based on organizational dynamics.

Despite the fact that the staff motivational engagement and incentive program is viewed as a proactive, preventive, and maintenance plan, most managers are still mired in focusing on cash bonuses, thinking they can solve a long-term, chronic organizational problem by using a short-term solution. Temporary fixes such as giving out cash bonuses with the expectation to induce behavioral change in employees have been known to be faulty and short-lived. They are known as sweeping the problem under the carpet, only for the same problem to resurface because its root cause was never addressed.

It is noteworthy that in staff motivation, what is convenient for the manager may be an inadequate satisfier for employees' needs. Besides, if staff incentive is applied only during an organizational downturn, it may create the perception in minds of employees that they are being manipulated to sign on to something designed only to benefit the organization. This is not only a recipe for employees' insubordination but an opportunity for them to question management ability to perform its duty.

Let's review an example whereby employees are repeatedly asked to do overtime or to report to work on their day off for extra cash bonus because of shortage of staff. Based on employees' reaction, there are three assumptions for management to take note of. If employees' answer is yes, are they doing so because they love the job itself, are they more interested in the cash bonus, or are they fearful that the boss might retaliate if they say no? For management to have a proper perspective on what creates employees' job satisfaction, it is important for them to study the difference between incentive and motivation. With regards to employees' on-the-job need satisfaction, incentive and motivation are not the same, but they are, however, found to reside on different sides of the same coin.

In an article titled "Incentive and Motivation—What's the Difference," it is written that even though the concept of incentive and motivation is not the same thing, "they tend to come hand in hand as one, but like a riddle, they don't work without each other and they are separate entities" (Wikipedia, 2020, para.1). Incentive is derived from external rewards that an employee receives for performing a job, while motivation is derived from the internal satisfaction an employee receives for loving the job he agrees to perform.

In an article titled "Incentive Vs. Motivation," Kaykas-wolff (2015) shines more light on the difference between incentive and motivation, stating:

> *Incentive means management gives you money when you do the kind of work they want but incentive will not necessarily produce the return on investment in terms of innovation, happiness, or stakeholder value . . . motivation means people do what they want to do in their work, where incentive*

*means people do whatever management wants and
pays them to do (Wikipedia 2020, para, 1–3).*

Some of the chronic organizational problems that a well-planned staff motivational engagement and incentive program seeks to prevent, needing long-term planning, may include shortage of staff, high absenteeism rate, lateness to work, low productivity rate, turnover rates, not meeting budget, to name a few. The negative findings resulting from an inappropriate application of the concept of incentive and motivation, or lack of understanding of their importance in employees' needs satisfaction thereof, is concerning, not only to the principle of holistic management but to what staff motivation represents.

Concurrently and in the main, holistic management and staff motivation advocate for staff cooperation, group morale, effective communication, connectivity, and optimization of all organizational parts, calling for the ability of all organizational members to be broad-minded and expansive in their thinking about their organizational well-being. This appears to be the important part of management to motivate employees to have a collective feeling of ownership and social stake-holding about and throughout the organization to enable them to focus, both on their personal well-being as well as the community well-being of the organization as a whole.

In an article titled "3 Critical Reasons Employees Become Unmotivated In The Workplace," Cole (2017) cited the three causes of unmotivated employees as "they don't feel connected to the successes of the company . . . they aren't given the opportunity to discover . . . they don't see the value" (Wikipedia 2020, para. 1–3).

Supervisory Management as a Factor in Employee Motivation in Nursing Homes

Staff supervision is an important part of a management function to ensure that company policies and standards are followed by staffers, and to ensure that they are kept motivated. Every staffer who is assigned a supervisor expects to be supervised, because a proper staff reward depends on proper supervision. At a minimum, people generally like to hear or know how well they are performing on their assignments and it sounds better when such an acknowledgment comes from their supervisors. The truth about human organization is that everyone needs some form of on-the-job supervision, more so in nursing homes, realizing the direct correlation that exists between the efficacy of supervision and the outcome of resident care. The importance of Benjamin Bloom's theory affecting human maturity in the method of teaching, learning, and the development of knowledge base was discussed in the preceding pages. Having an adequate knowledge base is a requirement for proper supervision.

The two main types of supervision that are frequently in use, consistent with the concept of Bloom taxonomy and requiring managers, especially those in nursing homes, to explore, are direct supervision and general supervision. Self-supervision describes individuals who tend to be highly skilled and mature, and therefore can self-supervise their work without any external support. In most management literatures, to be self-supervised also means to be unsupervised, whose applicability tends not to be grounded in McGregor's theory X about human nature or the nature of human organizations.

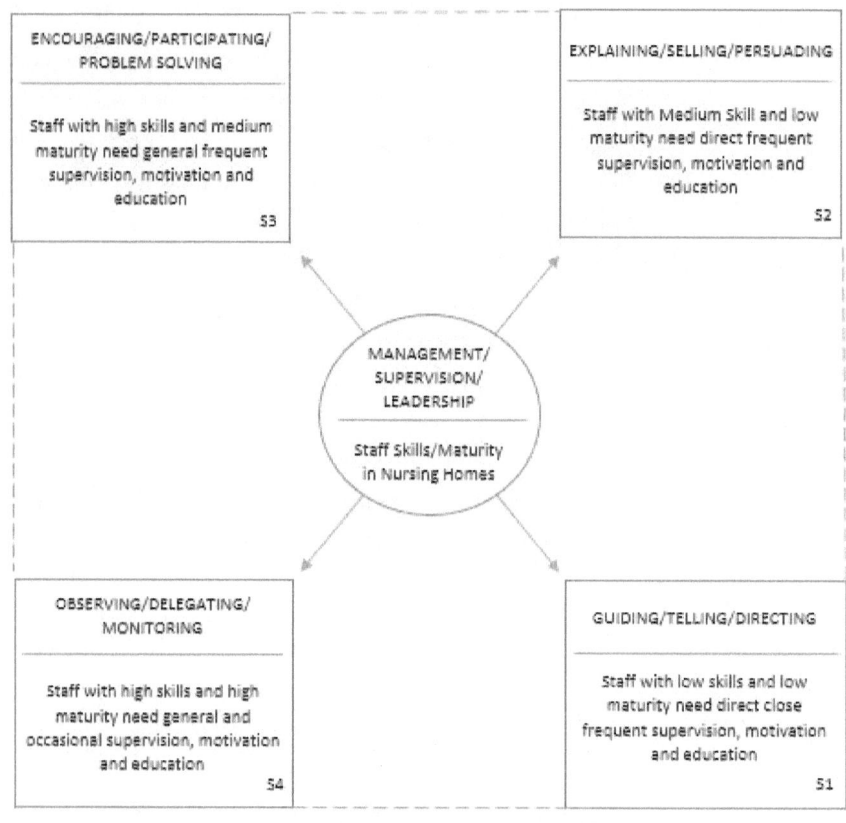

ENCOURAGING/PARTICIPATING/
PROBLEM SOLVING

Staff with high skills and medium
maturity need general frequent
supervision, motivation and
education
S3

EXPLAINING/SELLING/PERSUADING

Staff with Medium Skill and low
maturity need direct frequent
supervision, motivation and
education
S2

MANAGEMENT/
SUPERVISION/
LEADERSHIP

Staff Skills/Maturity
in Nursing Homes

OBSERVING/DELEGATING/
MONITORING

Staff with high skills and high
maturity need general and
occasional supervision, motivation
and education
S4

GUIDING/TELLING/DIRECTING

Staff with low skills and low
maturity need direct close
frequent supervision, motivation
and education
S1

Situational Leadership: Management/Supervision styles in
Holistic Nursing Home Management

Adapted from: Hersey et al (2001, 277) Management of
Organizational Behavior: Leading Human Resources, Eight
Edition, New Jersey, Prentice Hall, Inc.

Situational Leadership: Management/Supervisory Styles in Holistic Nursing Home Management

The theories of Bloom taxonomy in combination with Hersey/Blanchard situational leadership is designed to help managers, especially in nursing homes, in deciding adequate supervisory/management styles that meet organizational goals. For staff supervision to be adequate, especially in nursing homes, it requires physical observation, collection of data, evaluation, and redirection by a designated supervisor.

Bloom taxonomy is used to determine the maturity and skill levels in humans in the cognitive, affective, and sensory domains from low to high skill levels. Specific learning and achievement deficient needs are derived from the hierarchical taxonomy, ranging from knowing/remembering, understanding, applying, analyzing, evaluating, and creating. Even though Bloom taxonomy emanated from the academic environment, it has found relevance in assessing the skills and maturity levels of employees in order to determine work assignments and the level of supervision they would need.

Deciding the type of supervision to use varies and depends on the nature of the business organization and the error rate the organization is willing to risk resulting from poor supervision and quality assessment. Nursing homes can be regarded as high reliability organizations (HRO) because of their operational complexity, where the negative consequences of ineffective supervision and noncompliance can be significantly high, resulting in the public outcry.

In an article titled "5 Principles of a High Reliability Organization (HRO)," Jacobson (2019) defined HRO as "an organization that has succeeded in avoiding catastrophes despite a high level of risk and complexity" (Wikipedia, 2020, para 1).

In management practice, terminologies such as *manager, leader,* and supervisor are used to designate different job functions. While there are discernable dissimilarities in job functions, one role is explicitly common among them. In one form or another, they are all leaders, responsible not only for ensuring staff motivation but also assuring that organizational goals are met through their hierarchical supervisory roles, consistent within the context of positional and personal leadership.

In the totem pole of management hierarchy, supervisors are those who are closest to the production-line employees, assuring quality measures and employee motivation. In an article titled "The differences Between Leadership & Supervising," Kokemuller (2020) wrote: "management concepts of leadership and supervising have many similarities, but some important differences exist. In general, you can lead in many ways without being a supervisor, but good supervisors often have good leadership skills. Top managers often have good skills and effective supervisory skills" (Wikipedia, 2020, para. 1).

Several essential elements, personal qualifications, and responsibilities needed to become a supervisor or to improve supervisory skills are available for your reference, most of which are published in management journals or taught in business schools under supervisory management. Beyond assuring adequate production levels, the concept of employee supervision is to determine based on each employee's technical skill and social maturity levels how much supervision is needed to meet organizational goal, enhance employees' well-being and motivation, consisting of, but not limited to:

- Assisting employees in projects and case management
- Proving social and emotional support to employees—needs satisfaction
- Providing positive, effective feedback on job performance, assuring encouragement and constructive criticism
- Assuring positive mentoring relationship between employees and supervisor
- Creating and assuring positive work culture relating to ethno-cultural diversity and inclusion
- Assuring a fair and equitable handling of employees conflict resolution
- Providing professional training and development to employees consistent with their trades
- Assuring employees' manageable workloads and timely performance evaluations
- Providing employees with consistent and predictable assignments to ensure they remain emotionally connected to their job from start to finish, and vice versa.
- Providing enough employees that assures each employee's concentration on perfecting his/her assignment

- Determining how much supervision each level employee needs to ensure effectiveness in meeting organizational goal (see *Situational Leadership Model* by Hersey, Blanchard, and Johnson)
- Assuring equity in employee rewards and incentives

Referring to the above listed supervisory roles, it goes without saying that the job of being an effective supervisor, especially the first-line supervisor, is not easy. Whether you are in a manufacturing or service industry like healthcare, especially in nursing homes, the importance of the role that frontline supervisors and their employees play as the backbone of organizational success or failure cannot be overemphasized. It must be noted well that a dis-satisfier effect resulting in poor quality in nursing home organizations can manifest when there is a constant shortage of employees, when employees are shoveled around from one job assignment/station to another, when their workload is increased at short notice (Frederick Herzberg), and when the efficacy of the type of supervision used is undetermined. Nursing homes would benefit more when their supervisors have an unambiguous duty of providing direct close employee supervision, employee motivation, and minimizing causative factors of employees' dissatisfaction on the job, realizing that happy employees make productive employees.

Accordingly and with respect to supervisory leadership, Anita Roddick, cofounder of the Body Shop, is quoted, "what I have learned is that people become motivated when you guide them to the source of their own power and when you make heroes out of employees who personify what you want to see in the organization." And Steve Jobs of Apple is quoted, "my job is not to be easy on people . . . my job is to take these great people we have and push them and make them even better."

Supervision is a specific job designation where supervisors watch over the work of others. And by controlling it without doing it themselves, they are nevertheless held accountable, for better or for worse. In some organizations, such as in nursing homes, where employees tend to have the role of supervising others as part of their job description, the effectiveness of performing such dual responsibilities and being held accountable for both have remained questionable, especially in situations where achieving organizational goals require the separation of these job functions and direct supervision. Nursing homes can benefit from embracing a direct supervisory methodology, with an incumbent whose job description is only to supervise the work of others to proactively assure quality outcomes.

In most situations where an organization is not doing well—such as experiencing low productivity level or service inadequacy—it is usually caused by what is happening within the rank and file. Whenever an employee or a group of employees is dissatisfied about something, it calls for a supervisor's intervention within the open-door policy of openness and transparency between management and employees.

Over the years, the military has seemed to have a better understanding than its civilian counterpart of the importance of taking care of its rank and file if the mission of winning a war is to be achieved. And in the case of a civilian enterprise, if the organizational goal is to be achieved. Consequently, when organizations miss their mark, prudent supervisors should find it best to start their corrective investigations with the rank and file to see why they are less motivated, efficient, or productive. Being a supervisor calls for a duty to care for workers to ensure that their emotional, personal, and material needs are satisfied. According to an article published by the Jeanne M. Holm Center titled "Effective Supervision," "being the effective supervisor will demand a great deal of time and attention. Supervision is a continual, rather than periodic task; you're never 'done' supervising" (Wikipedia, 2020, para.25).

As we emphasized earlier, frontline supervisors are a part of management, who are different from the working class but with a function of playing an intermediary role between management and workers to prevent workers from being disgruntled and taking a unilateral action against management. The demand from the working class (proletariat) for fair treatment from management (bourgeoisie) started shortly after the Industrial Revolution of the 1760s. Karl Marx (1818–1883) had a disdain for the powerlessness of the working class as he viewed the working conditions of factories as terrible. Consequently, his philosophy of the "dictatorship of the proletariat," even though directed toward those who held political powers in society in that era, also had implications in criticizing how the British working class were treated in the hands of management, resulting in the formation of the labor union movement of the early eighteenth century.

In the United States, unionism has been active since the 1850s as an option for workers' action if they are not treated fairly by management. It is also noteworthy that in today's economy this hidden power of the rank and file employees, though seldom discussed or openly recognized by management, still exists, to include surreptitious sabotage of organizational goals or forming a workers' union to bargain for wages, benefits, and better working conditions.

As we have repeatedly stated, one of the functions of management/supervisor is to assure the welfare of employees, to ensure high staff morale and motivation. Whenever management's ineptitude abounds in the workplace, it encourages not only the existence of workers' unions but also their momentum in opposition to management to correct the malpractice as perceived by employees. As management would like to be the only king on the hill, the welcoming of workers' unions is more likely than not to be rare, and in most human resources literature, the struggle for power, legitimacy, and conflicts between management and workers' unions has been well documented.

Rubin (1960), in his article titled "A Theory of Conflict and Power in Union-Management Relations," wrote: "two concepts are almost universally used by analysts of union-management relations. The first is that of conflict; the second is power" (Wikipedia, 2020, para. 1). As discussed in preceding pages of this book, there is a simple solution to maintaining equanimity and fair play in today's workplace that doesn't lie in the power of workers' unions or management totalitarianism, but in the holistic management approach and its advocacy for employee motivation, welfare, and the inclusion of all organizational members as stakeholders, not only to eliminate workplace conflicts between workers and management but also workers' unions.

Eight-Hour Workday: Implication in Holistic Nursing Home Management and Nursing Home Quality

The goal of holistic nursing home management is to ensure an improved care and caring for the residents by alert and oriented staff, and to fish out negative factors that could pose impediments to achieving that goal. The eight-hour workday is a universal law with a long history from which the concept of overtime work is based. Historically, in 1593, Phillip II, king of Spain (1527–1598) established an eight-hour workday that became a universal standard in 1919. During the Industrial Revolution, it was Robert Owen (1771–1858) who advocated a ten-hour workday to include recreational time and rest. In the same period, Karl Max's (1818–1883) advocacy for the working class was also linked to long hours of work as part of poor working conditions with negative implication on the health and well-being of workers.

In 1866, the Knight of Labor in the United States demanded that an eight-hour workday be enacted into law by the Congress, but this demand lingered and only became law in 1940 due to the advocacy of both owners and management of Ford Motors and General Motors in the mid-1930s. In 2016, the 1919 original eight-hour workday initiated by Phillip II was ratified by the International Labor Union, and remains the universal labor law.

In the United States and Europe, working long hours, a.k.a. overtime, has become a conventional thing to do but may not be the right thing to do in some work situations. There are advantages and disadvantages in overtime work for both the employer and the employee. However, there is a need to use an entirely different lens in evaluating the advantages and disadvantages of employee overtime in health care settings, especially in nursing homes. Because overtime is often warranted due to shortage of labor or management miscalculation in increased demand for product and services, investing at the front end for growth and development in skilled labor force makes a better sense than incurring overtime cost. Besides, there are research studies that correlate employees' overtime with employees' stress, fatigue, decreased attention span, burnout, decreased productivity, increased turnover rates, and absenteeism. Employees' productivity is known to inversely decline with overtime. The metrics frequently used by researchers to show the impact of overtime on productivity is a 10 percent increase in overtime resulting in a 2.4 percent decrease in productivity.

The nature of a nursing home operation is to care for the sick and the elderly, for which its employees must embrace the concept of being "alert and oriented" as it is meant to apply in the health care setting. In most work situations, employees who perform critical and sensitive work are considered to be "alert and oriented" after they must have had a minimum of eight hours sleep or rest. Nursing home employees are required to remain quick, vigilant, and well trained to respond to any unusual circumstances affecting the residents. In recent years, most state regulators in nursing homes have increased nursing staffing ratios, which are normally described as hours per patient day (HPPD), despite the lack of a proportional growth in the number of nurses entering the profession. Consequently, whenever there is staff shortage due to callouts or no one to hire, the only option left to fulfill the regulatory staffing ratio mandate is to ask any available staff to work overtime to create a "phantom of sufficient staffing." If staff are already stressed, burnt out, and lacking attention after having worked a full shift on the first job or the second job, their ability to adequately provide residents' care can be reduced/nonexistent, and their continuous presence on the job can become a contributor to poor quality of care and a decrease in nursing home quality, confirming that HPPD is a quantitative, budgetary-based assumption and not a qualitative assumption of employees' productivity or efficiency.

In an article titled "Nursing Overtime: The Good, The Bad, The OMG," Learning (2018) wrote to confirm a study showing that "as nursing overtime increased, so did patient dissatisfaction with care. What's more, burnout, job dissatisfaction and an intention to leave the job were more than twice as likely among nurses who worked shifts of 10 hours or longer than nurses who worked shorter shifts" (Wikipedia, 2020, para 11). Consequently, an eight-hour workday is not only an ideal assumption that protects workers' health and well-being, but also an assurance that increases workers' productivity, interpreted as increased quality of care for the residents in nursing homes. In a study of nurses work hours and adverse events titled "The Effect of Work Hours on Adverse Events and Errors in Health Care," Olds and Clarke (2011) concluded that "all of the adverse event or error variables were related to working more than 40 hours in the average workweek" (Wikipedia, 2020, para 3). In this study, specific errors were found in needle stick, nosocomial infection, patient falls with injury, and medication errors.

Ultimately, by using cost-benefit analysis, owners of nursing homes would need to develop a strategic plan to address nurse shortages in their place of business; at a minimum, the shortage of CNAs, who provide 80–90 percent of the direct care and felt needs in nursing homes. It is time to do more toward improving nursing home quality and the issue of nurse shortages as there appears to be room for improvement.

Chapter 14

Understanding Behavior Science Management and the Concept of Teaming Up with the Masters

The purpose of this chapter is first and foremost to promote the merits of a lifelong learning for all organizational members, especially for health care workers in nursing homes. Holistic management requires the ability of managers, and indeed workers, to adapt to new approaches in managing organizations to meet new demands. Supervising others or dabbling into behavior management requires a formal education, the right kind of leadership training, and continuous learning from the works of past and present behavior scientists for guidance in what we call "teaming up with the masters."

Why? Managing the behavior of others in an organization can be complex, especially when a specific organizational outcome is expected. Going alone is not only primitive but also a layman's approach to management. Also, depending on the residual knowledge from our past classroom learning may not be good enough in a dynamic and changing work environment. In most organizations like nursing homes, it is already a regulatory requirement that employees obtain continuing education units (CEUs) for their clinical or managerial practice. The main purpose of embarking on extramural or CEU courses we envisage has been for employees to update their knowledge base. It is advisable, therefore, that employees examine their prerequisite knowledge in the subject area that will enable them to intellectually benefit from taking the course.

It is also noteworthy that the value-added effect of on-the-job-training does not come from acquiring the CEUs in and of themselves or merely fulfilling the regulatory requirement, but from assuring the meaning to what was learned relative to change and on-the-job effectiveness. Secondly, we are reminding managers and leaders of organizations that their management style can hold the key toward an effective leadership, and that the management styles they adopt be drawn from the philosophies and concepts of scholars whose work have been proven credible, worthy, and successful. Because management is science capable of producing a cause-and-effect result—facts, not fiction—we decry management by "shooting in the dark." And because holistic management is a decision-making enterprise, "shooting from the hip" decisions can be likened to playing a game of chance, devoid of producing the desired outcome, heuristic value, or replication. Some of these theoretical frameworks are listed in the succeeding pages for current and future business managers to review and to update their management skills.

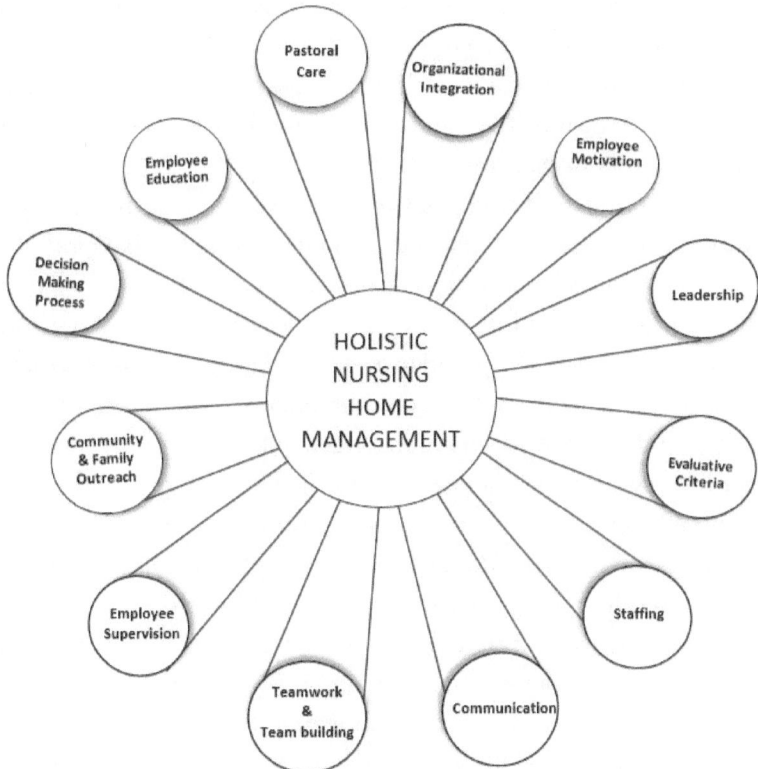

Conceptual View in Holistic NH Management

In most religions like the Catholic faith, believers have patron saints to consult in times of need. In the behavioral science field, there are many renowned behavior theorists who can be regarded, if not as saints, but as our patrons based on their behavioral science doctrines, philosophies, theories, and concepts available to learn from and use as applicable. Our schools of management in colleges and universities are traditionally designed for andragogic teaching and learning of these scientific thoughts, theories, philosophies, and concepts, in which the learner's intrinsic motivation is important in order for him to achieve his personal growth and development.

There are two types of learning techniques available to business managers and organizational leaders whose interest is to acquire new knowledge and skills or improve on the existing ones. Experiential learning is learning by reflecting on the business or personal actions or decisions we took in order to make necessary correction. In academic learning, the learner can resort to a classroom-based teaching or acquire needed information from secondary sources, which are usually scholarly books and articles created by someone else. In most cases, learners in management science can list and study the philosophies and theories of selected authors that are applicable to their interest.

It was previously noted that in management training, potential managers are involved in exploring management and behavioral science theories under the broad subject areas of organizational development, management development, and psychology. Essentially, in organizational development, trainees are exposed to a science-based process of structuring and designing organizations to achieve an effective operation with built-in capacities for change. Whereas in management development, trainees are exposed to a systematic science-based process of acquiring knowledge, skills, and attitudes suitable in managing workers in order for them to be motivated and productive. Management development training comes with the expectation that the learner will not only master the subject materials from secondary sources or in a classroom setting, but will be able to apply them in real-life situations to achieve organizational goals, which include improved employee supervision and motivation.Psychology can be defined as the scientific study and understanding of the human mind, its functions and behavior relating to persons, place, time, or thing.

Human motivation and behavior are by and large determined by human needs, desires, and wants that are available in the external environment, provided independently or by others. Needs, desires, and wants in humans are deemed to be either satisfied or unsatisfied, necessitating the presence or absence of homeostasis. Motive is the reason why a particular human action is taken control of by the level of his psychological or physiological arousal.

The theory of human motivation is coined from the word *motive*, and is designed as an equalizer between the human beings and their needs satisfaction. Management theories are inseparably theories of human motivation used to define how human behaviors can be adequately managed under certain environmental conditions so that human beings can be successful in their daily activities. Because scientific theories are factual information derived from tested hypothesis, they are made available to guide and enlighten readers and practitioners in managing all aspects of our practical life, including the lives of others existing under the spheres of our influence, responsibility, and authority.

In an article titled "Just a Theory: 7 Misused Science Words," Ghose (2013) confirmed that "a scientific theory is an explanation of some aspect of the natural world that has been substantiated through experiments and testing" (Wikipedia, 2020, para. 3). In another article, titled "What Is a Scientific Theory," Bradford (2017) explained and wrote "most people use the word theory to mean an idea or hunch that someone has, but in science the theory refers to the way that we interpret facts" (Wikipedia, 2020, para. 1). Applied scientific theory is defined as using the existing scientific knowledge to solve new management and human behavior problems we face.

As relevant as these scientific theories have become as frames of reference in managing human behavior, the necessity to routinely review these theorists and their historic contributions has become unavoidable as well. Most of the contributions made to behavior science, management, and human motivation by such principal theorists as Abraham Maslow, Elton Mayo, Paul Hershey, Kenneth Blanchard, Dewey Johnson, and others have already been discussed in the preceding pages. A few other behavior science theorists we have identified as "masters" in management science and employee motivation practice, and worthy of review by managers and organizational leaders, include, but are not limited to, B. F. Skinner, Sigmund Freud, Karen Horney, Chris Argyris, Frederick Herzberg, Douglas McGregor, William Ouchi, Victor Vroom, F. E. Fiedler, David McClelland, and Herbert A. Simon. These listed theorists and their work, dating back decades, if not centuries, are recognized to be relevant as a foundation for holistic management practice. It can therefore be concluded that when practitioners in their different fields of endeavor understudy and inculcate notable behavior science theories in their work, they are imperceptibly emulating the theorists themselves by applying their philosophies to improve the overall quality of societal life for them and others. For example, people who engage in the study of the New Testament Bible would say they want to be Christlike, whereas those who choose to study Peter Drucker or Allan Savory would say they want to have an understanding of their popular concepts of "management by objective" or "holistic management" in business management respectively.

In economics, economists who practice the economic doctrine of John Maynard Keynes (1883–1946) of governmental involvement in national economy are called the Keynesians, differentiating them from those who follow Friedrich A. Von Hayek (1899–1992) or Adam Smith's (1723–1790) doctrine of governmental non-interference.

In medical and nursing science, it is not uncommon to invoke the guidance of Hippocrates and Florence Nightingale respectively, or Avedis Donabedian (1919–2000), known as the father of quality assurance in health care. In philosophy, ethics, and morality, we read and adopt the worldview of Aristotle, Plato, Socrates, and Cicero, to name a few.

Acquiring and applying empirical and scientific knowledge to manage present or predict future situations, even as we fend through life, is not only normative but also one in which the interpretation and propagation of the meaning and purpose of education, especially adult education, is based. When John Dewey (1859–1952) stated that "education is not preparation for life; education is life itself," he was referring to education as a lifelong process and as an agent of social change.

In an article titled "What's the Purpose of Education in the 21st Century?" Strauss (1915) shed more light on the purpose of education, and saw it as preparing people for "life, work and citizenship . . . and how people live in the world is critical to all three purposes of education. Critical thinking, creativity, interpersonal skills and a sense of social responsibility all influence success in life, work and citizenship" (Wikipedia, 2020, para. 4). It is noteworthy that the more we become clients to these scientific theorists and perceive them as our therapists or invisible mentors, the more the transference and countertransference of knowledge will enhance our best practices.

In psychotherapy, it is the presence of the transference and countertransference between clients and therapists that creates a meaningful partnership toward wellness. Because behaviorism is the essence of management, we similarly expect managers and leaders who study, embrace, and apply the philosophies and theories of the behavior science theorists to receive the benefits of improving their management skills, achieving organizational goals, and investing in management behaviors and practice that can be repeated with some amount of exactitude.

In a book titled *The Human Nature of Organizations*, Brown (1973, 164) evaluated the importance of education in human organizations as a means of developing organizational leaders to acquire the knowledge base they need, not only to sustain organizations but also to manage change, stating:

> *Knowledge is a means rather than the end . . . a potential leader should develop a sense of history that the future grows out of the past. This includes the ability, through the study of many periods and areas of history—cultural, political, and social—to sense and understand the basic factors in change which often lie beneath the surface, but which gain momentum over time . . . a sense of history helps one to gain perspective and to see the vital distinction between the conservation of a principle and a change in the appropriate method to conserve that principle . . .*

The theorists and their theoretical frameworks presented below are mere synoptic samples among many others intended for practitioners to learn from with in-depth studies, remembering what Isaac Newton (1642–1726/27) admittedly stated, "if I have seen further than others, it is by standing upon the shoulders of giants," and "to me there has never been a higher source of earthly honor or distinction than that connected with advances in science."

These important philosophical thoughts do not only affirm important worldviews on the efficacy of science and their patronage, but also shines more light on the article titled "Bad Management Theories are Destroying Good Management Practices." In this article, Ghoshal (n d) wrote on the future direction of science, the need to interpret and use applied science carefully, and affirmed how scientific "theories influence practice and managers adopt theorists' worldview" (Wikipedia, 2020, para 12). Over the years, these are some of the theorists in behavior science who are known for imagining the world we now live in, and creating different platforms for change so that human beings can live better in the future:

A study of B. F. Skinner (1904–1990) reveals that he theorized the concept of "reinforcement" to help managers in managing acceptable and unacceptable human behaviors. Defining reinforcement as a mechanism of strengthening behavior, Skinner went on to differentiate between positive and negative reinforcement as a form of human intervention to continue a favorable human behavior or discontinue the unfavorable ones, respectively. Today, the concept of reinforcement is not only popular among managers in workplace behavior management but also in classroom management for teachers, and even in the parental management of children in the home. His operant conditioning concept, a.k.a. instrumental conditioning, is also known to be helpful when humans can learn and achieve behavior change through understanding reward and punishment mechanisms.

Sigmund Freud (1856–1936) focused his psychoanalytical theory on human personality, directing our attention, among others, to anxiety neurosis in humans. He saw human psyche as inherently comprising of the id, ego, and superego, in which there must a balance to avoid poor quality of life. In the psychic apparatus, the role of the superego—which has two parts: the ego ideal and conscience—are learned behaviors that must be taught beginning at the early stages of human development. They are the internalized ideals and moral aptitudes that individuals acquire from parents, society, and others in authority. The ego ideals are the rules and standards set by those in authority, which describes what constitute good behavior. While conscience represents rules that describe what constitute bad behaviors that generate guilt if there is a breach of conduct and when behavioral boundaries are crossed. The lesson we learn from the Freudian psychic apparatus is that in our societies, workplaces, educational systems, and political systems, we need citizens who are psychologically well, know right from wrong, to be productive members of society.

Karen Horney (1885–1952) is known as a protégé of Sigmund Freud who was responsible for neo-Freudianism. Like Freud, Karen was also concerned about human neurosis, but unlike Freud, she saw human neurosis to be continuous and sporadic throughout one's lifetime, resulting from basic human anxieties inherent in our interpersonal relationships, citing our attitudes as we relate toward self and others. As documented in her concept of "neurotic trends," human interaction for conflict resolution depends on our attitudes toward people from whom we are either moving away, moving against, moving toward. We see people moving toward one another as being consistent with holistic management that produces teamwork. She went on to develop another important concept she called ten patterns of "neurotic needs" relating to human needs for affection, social recognition, love of problem-solving partners, and so on.

Chris Argyris (1923–2013), known as a cofounder of the concept of organizational development, has made great contributions to management and behavior science. Argyris advocated that to achieve high productivity in organizations, managers must treat employees positively and as responsible adults who are usually willing and interested in carrying more responsibilities and participating in the company's decision-making process. He theorized the concept of a "single-loop learning" and a "double-loop learning" in problem-solving situations—personal or organizational. According to Argyris, a single-loop learning in organization occurs when organizational problems are examined superficially or suppressed only for them to reoccur. Organizational problems that are thoroughly investigated not only to achieve permanent resolution but also to achieve non-reoccurrence is the double-loop learning approach.

Frederick Herzberg' (1923–2000) motivator-hygiene theory, a.k.a. two-factor theory, has been useful in designing employee motivational programs that affect employees' morale and productivity. Herzberg, in his theory of motivator versus hygiene factors, identified causes of employees' workplace satisfaction and dissatisfaction respectively. According to Herzberg, motivating factors, a.k.a. job satisfiers, such as achievement, recognition, the work itself, responsibility, advancement, and growth, have intrinsic values responsible for causing not only employees' workplace satisfaction but also high productivity. Hygiene factors, a.k.a. job dis-satisfiers, such as company policies, supervision, relationship with supervisor and peers, salary, status, and job security, have extrinsic values capable of causing employees' workplace dissatisfaction that is not enough cause for employees' resignation and so forth, but oftentimes enough reason to stall productivity.

Douglas McGregor (1906–1964) is well known for theorizing theory X and Y as contained in his publication titled *The Human Side of Enterprise.* The impact of theory X and Y is strongly felt in the area of supervisory management and employee motivation. McGregor's theory identified for management that in a given workforce there are potentially two types of employees. There are those identified as theory X employees and those identified as theory Y employees. The assumption of theory X is that some human beings instinctively dislike to work and therefore must be tightly supervised. Theory Y assumption is that some human beings who, beyond liking to work, are self-directed and prefer a collaborative supervisory relationship. McGregor then went on to list six characteristics of theory X employees and five characteristics of theory Y employees to help managers adjust their management/supervisory styles accordingly.

William Ouchi (1943–present) theorized theory Z as an additional factor to McGregor's theory X and Y. The main tenet of theory Z was a focus on increasing employee loyalty to the company as a means of increasing job satisfaction and productivity. Ouchi's theory Z went on to advocate that companies provide not only lifetime jobs for employees but also assure their well-being on and off the job. Theory Z also emphasized the importance of employees' relationship with their employers that creates a partnership between them and other employees, clearly suggestive of employee teamwork and a participative management/supervisory style. Noteworthy in theory Z is that being of Japanese descent, this theorist was also American educated and who was treading between two cultures in his approach to management in the 1980s when the American economy was performing worse than the Japanese economy. Theory Z has eight characteristics that should be well noted, especially as in-job rotation with preference to employing generalists instead of specialists.

Victor Vroom (1932–present) is known for using his expectancy theory to explain employees' motivation with regards to management behavior. Expectancy theory is the assumption that employees who perform work are operating in their best self-interest, trust, and faith, and believe that the reward they will receive from management will meet their perceived expectations. In this sense, it becomes important that in order for management to fully meet employees' satisfaction they must carefully evaluate and identify employees' needs, endeavor to provide rewards that meets individuals' value, set goals for employees that are achievable, and ensure that their rewards equate their effort and are delivered when earned.

According to Vroom, the three components of expectancy theory to generate employee motivation when present are as follows: expectancy, instrumentality, and valence, or expectancy + instrumentality + valence =

employee motivation. Expectancy represents the belief employees have that the desired outcome will be achieved if they work harder. Instrumentality represents the belief employees have that their reward will be accorded them when the desired outcome is achieved. And valence represents the value of the reward employees associate with the expected outcome. In expectancy theory, management behavior and action are effective when they are contemplated from employees' perspective, perception, and expectation.

Fred Fiedler (1922–2017) is recognized for his research works in industrial and organizational psychology, notably the path-goal theory, situational leadership, and decision-making theories. His contingency theory, which focused on leadership styles, maintained that there is "no one best way" in leading people, and that different situations demand different leadership style. The implication of the contingency theory is that leaders/managers can only be successful if they can match their leadership styles to the situational factors. In this case, most hiring managers could benefit from the contingency theory, which requires the matching of the right people to the right job in accordance with the job demands. This is to say that hiring a college professor to teach kindergarten would not be a good match.

Fiedler is considered as a forerunner of Hershey and Blanchard, who later theorized the situational leadership demanding leaders/managers to be flexible and eclectic in their management styles to be able to adapt and respond to different situational factors within the organization. Noteworthy to leaders/managers also is their understanding of the similarity and difference between the contingency theory and the situational leadership theory. Both theories are similar because of their emphasis on the importance of situational variations within organizations, but differ in that both have different leadership demands and expectations.

David McClelland (1917–1998) is known for his expectancy value theory of motivation, a.k.a. achievement motivation theory, consisting of three human needs for affiliation, achievement, and power. McClelland went on to describe these needs as "acquired," meaning they don't exist permanently in people because they are culturally and experientially developed. Affiliation needs reflect people who can thrive well when part of a work group where they can socialize, establish relationships with others to be loved and accepted. Achievement needs reflect people with strong desire to work hard to master their job and excel in what they do, preferring high-risk situations to low-risk situations. Power needs reflect people who are motivated by the need to control and influence others, with status and recognition being important to them.

McClelland's theory is believed to be beneficial in a corporate setting to select organizational members in the areas of work that they are best suited. McClelland, a follower of Henry Murray (1893–1988), is recognized for developing the following personality assessment instruments: the thematic appreciation test, the behavior event interview, and the test of thematic analysis—all of which are used in job interviews to select candidates for employment.

Herbert A. Simon (1916–2001) is known for his contribution to management science, specializing in the theory of decision-making. He defined decision-making as a rational process of identifying the problem, collecting all available information relative to the problem, establishing the goal and evaluation criteria. However, his theories of "bounded rationality," "satisficing," and "intractability," dating back to 1957, are profound, not only in understanding the importance of personal or organizational decision-making but also what goes into making effective decisions.

In bounded rationality, Simon explains the limitations that can exist to prevent decision makers from optimizing their decisions. His theory of satisficing explains the why and how decision makers may sometimes have to settle with less than the best decisions they can make. Intractability is defined as a problem that can occur in the decision-making process. Even though these intractability problems do exist during the decision-making process, ranging from the limitation in human cognitive ability, available time, available information, mental capability, and other materials, they are not a foregone conclusion in preventing decision makers from not seeking maximizing rather than satisficing their decisions.

According to Allan Savory, decision-making is essential in holistic management, making Simon's theories noteworthy for practitioners and students of holistic management. Simon is also known as one of founding fathers of artificial intelligence, who rightly predicted that by 1965 "machines will be capable of doing any work a man can do." In an article titled "Herbert Simon, Innovation, and Heuristics," Kheirandish and

Mousavi (2019) documented one of Simon's 1957 arguments relating to managing organizations, stating that "in order to survive in a changing business arena, executives are charged with designing organizational environments conducive to innovation" (Wikipedia 2020, para 3).

Chapter 15

Summary, Comments, and Recommendations

The history of the present-day nursing home organizations is traceable to the tenth-century English almshouses built and managed for the purpose of caring for poor and destitute people. In the United States of America, the psychological impact of the concept of public poorhouse that was adopted in the 1600s is still felt in today's nursing homes.

There is no sufficient information on how the services provided in these public poorhouses were paid for, but long after the emergence of nursing homes from the concept of the poorhouse in the United States, care conditions continued to remain deplorable. Accordingly, governmental involvement was inevitable through the Social Security Act of 1935, a.k.a. Old Age Assistance program, which provided only the institutionalized public poor housing but not financial support to pay for personal needs of individuals who lived in these "public poorhouses." Today, the majority of institutionalized people in US nursing homes are sponsored by Medicaid as enacted in 1965.

The Medicaid program is defined as a government-sponsored welfare program whose beneficiaries must be poor, destitute, and in need of custodial care. The period after Medicaid was followed by a slow paced and incremental quality improvement through privatization and myriad government regulations on nursing homes. All things considered, the Omnibus Budget Reconstruction Act of 1987 (OBRA '87) has been credited for establishing a uniform standard of care and a monitoring system that is applicable to all nursing facilities throughout the United States. However, it must be noted that despite OBRA '87, the general negative perception about these institutions and the people who live there has remained almost the same as they were in the almshouse/poorhouse days. The negative psychosocial effect of living in a nursing facility, as well as what shapes the negative perception of the public about people who lived there is undeniable, needing further research, but one that must change.

In a thesis titled "The Contempt of the Poor: A Closer Look into New York City Almshouse in the Nineteenth Century and the Treatment of the Lower Class," Jenney (2019) defined contempt to mean "those living in poverty were deemed worthless in society . . . that the upper class was seen as the only population worthy of happiness and prosperity, especially compared to those experiencing poverty" (Wikipedia, 2020, para.1, 3). In much of our literature reviews, it is revealed that many people are asking the same questions about the problem of nursing home quality. Also, there are research studies still showing the public apathy toward nursing home residency for which a dichotomy tends to exist between the psychological rejection based on the concept of the almshouse and the need for an appreciable improvement in nursing home quality. According to the National Citizens' Coalition for Nursing Home Reform (NCCNHR) article titled "The Nurse Staffing Crisis in Nursing Homes," and endorsed by several organizations, Menio et al. (2001) listed some of the causative factors for nurse shortages in nursing homes needing change as recruiting and hiring qualified job applicants, retention, payment systems, wage and benefits, education, training and supervision, workload, philosophy of the organizational/staff empowerment, workplace safety, opportunities for advancement, external issues such as transportation and child care, and public perception, and wrote:

> *A negative public perception of nursing home care and caregiving has also been cited as a contributing factor to the staffing crisis . . . however, the undersigned organizations believe that*

the crisis can be alleviated or resolved by changes in our public policies, professional practices, and education (Wikipedia 2020, para 13, 14)

Besides the urgent need for a psychosocial reorientation on the public's perception of nursing homes and a review of the above recommendations by Menio, our observation is that nursing homes by nature have too many moving and unintegrated parts for government regulations alone to fix. There is a tendency that these longstanding organizational dis-satisfiers in nursing homes are either being normalized or the management of these institutions is desensitized about them. A dis-satisfier is defined as a working condition that may cause an employee to quit or become unmotivated and unproductive. There is also the tendency for nursing home practitioners and stakeholders alike to oversimplify the management operations in nursing homes rather than acknowledge the complexities that rightly characterizes it in order to find appropriate solutions to the problems of nursing home quality. For example, for so long, nursing staff shortages have been blamed more for lack of nursing home quality than any of the issues listed in the NCCNHR report.

While others received lip service toward nursing home quality, there tends to be no plan to address these concerns holistically. The direct link existing between shortage of staff (CNAs) and poor nursing home quality is undeniable. CNAs are the backbone of nursing home care. The fact that we aren't producing enough of them and their salaries aren't high enough to retain them on one job, nursing homes are enhancing their ineffectiveness when they split jobs to make ends meet or when they are assigned to care for too many resident per shift.

The problem of staff shortages relating to the lack of nursing home quality is also seen to be aggravated by such issues as lack of effective direct staff supervision, the current approach to management functions, inappropriate response to employee job dissatisfaction, and the implication of the public perception of nursing homes in general, all of which are competing factors. The concept of the dignity of labor implies human self-esteem emanating from employees working in an organization where the work they do is respected, perceived by them and others as important. An employee's self-esteem is linked to an observable or reported success or failure in achieving an organizational goal.

In an industry like nursing homes where the definition of nursing home quality can be amorphous despite OBRA's quality standard, and in part depending on how an individual resident or family feels and interprets it, there nevertheless tends to exist a direct relationship between the satisfying of residents' needs and achieving employees' self-esteem needs that has so far remained elusive. To achieve residents' needs satisfaction, nursing home quality and employees' self-esteem, there is need to reevaluate how supervisory management is conducted in nursing homes.

The main tenet of holistic nursing home management is that all parts of the nursing home organization and its organizational issues such as those posed by NCCNHR as far back as 2001 be strongly integrated into one manageable whole and supervised proactively. Thomas Reid (1710–1796) maintained that "the chain is only as strong as its weakest link." The importance of an effective resident and staff supervision is to proactively identify and correct the weak links in the system having the potential to cause harm to the residents.

The nursing home operational reform, which has been traditionally looked at from a clinical nursing perspective, has been insufficient. In order to obtain and maintain compliance, a new round of nursing home reform reflecting holistic management principles is needed in the managerial skills for planning, organizing, coordinating, controlling, leading, supervising, staffing, staff motivation, and decision-making and adopting the conceptual view in holistic nursing home management, which nurses alone cannot provide.

As implicated in the holistic management approach, nursing home organizations need a new management approach, know-how, and a process of bringing together all the affected parts and issues in nursing homes. Like any broken-down car, we need a mechanic with new tools and the understanding of its parts, how the parts and issues are connected, and how to bring them together in order to fix the car and make it run. When car manufacturers decided to modernize cars by computerizing them, there was a commensurate retraining of auto mechanics who would repair and maintain them.

In an article titled "An Assessment of Strategies for Improving Quality of Care in Nursing Homes," Wiener (2003) observed that "despite substantial regulatory oversight, quality of care in nursing homes remains problematic" (Wikipedia, 2020, para. 1). In this article, Wiener pointed out several strategies that nursing home organizations can take internally to improve quality of care, and added that:

> *Although the previous strategies rely on forces outside nursing homes to either force nursing homes to improve quality of care or to provide incentives to do so, a strong argument can be made that nursing homes themselves must take responsibility to improve quality of care (Wikipedia 2020, para. 37).*

In another article, titled "The Challenges of Improving Nursing Home Quality," Konetzka (2020) posed the question "why are solutions to low-quality nursing home care so elusive?" (Wikipedia, 2020, para.3). While the findings in these articles are worth noting, they represent the same unresolved problems and hence a demand to rethink new ways to solve the problems of nursing home quality instead of "beating the same dead horse." Rethinking business management approach in the era of change does not only apply to nursing homes but also to all types of business organizations seeking to survive well. An article titled "The Time Has Come for Holistic Business Strategy Solis" (2011) posed two important questions: "What's the biggest problem in business today?" "What is the solution?" And wrote the answer as follows:

> I believe we need to fundamentally rethink the closely held tenets of business strategy, especially in light of the geopolitical and environmental situation we now face. To put it simply, it is time for organizations large or small to adopt a holistic business strategy that empowers more employees to think about the whole of the business; to more fully understand the ins and outs of the product/service offering; and ultimately focus on serving their

markets instead of serving the stock market (Wikipedia, 2020, para.1).

Holistic Management in the Era of Change: A Pathway to a Sustainable Nursing Home Quality is written to bring the concept, philosophy, and framework of holistic management to the forefront of business management, especially in nursing homes. The goal of holistic management as presented herewith does not suggest a replacement of classicism and humanism as management philosophies, but to provide the expansion they need in modernizing management practice that reflects change.

In medicine and nursing, Hippocrates and Nightingale appealed to the holistic care of patients. Holistic business management is intended to enhance evidence-based practice in management functions, allowing for all organizational activities to be holistically evaluated. Unlike in holistic medical and nursing practice where the concept of evaluating and treating of the whole person—body, mind, spirit, culture, socioeconomic background and environment—has already taken root, evidence-based practice in holistic business management functions is still elusive due to the limitation in human factors and managerial coordination that are needed to optimize outcomes.

In holistic business management, it is no longer sufficient to base a successful organization on financial statements or shareholders' equity alone. In accordance with holistic management principles, more attention has to be directed to the qualitative aspects of the organization as they relate to human needs and how the organizational systems are interconnected. Consequently, the twelve concepts of holistic management, which emphasize and represent the new standard of measurement for evaluating organizational effectiveness, have been sufficiently discussed. They are organizational integration, decision-making process, developing a culture of teamwork and teambuilding, developing effective bottom-up lines of communication, leadership, pastoral care, staffing needs, employee motivation, employee supervision, employee education, evaluative criteria, and community and family outreach.

From the perspective of holistic nursing home management, the rule of thumb should be if something is purported to exist, it should not be treated as nonexistent or unimportant. Focusing on the twelve main concepts of holistic management is intended to help managers, especially nursing home managers, to gain and maintain a broader perspective on what is required to keep their organizations fully functional and productive.

The evolution of holistic management from the scientific/classical and humanistic management approaches is its introduction as a "value-based decision-making framework that integrates all aspects of planning for social, economic, and environmental considerations" (Wikipedia, 2020, para.2). The importance of an effective decision-making in an organization, hitherto not highlighted in the classical management approach, as one of the functions of management or as its main function has been sufficiently discussed in the previous pages of this edition.

Holistic management was initially regarded as a management principle for agri-business, deriving its motivation and subsequent success within the process of decision-making that is now widely applied to other businesses as well. Reportedly "there are many benefits to companies using holistic approaches. It allows them to see which sections of the company are failing or are weaker compared to others" (Wikipedia, 2020, para 2). Understanding and applying holistic management in the workplace demands hard work and managerial vigilance but with higher payoff return on investment. Nursing homes, for example, can avoid a cyclical underperformance and unplanned hospitalizations of residents by using a holistic management approach, not only within their functional departments but also in direct resident care.

Holism is defined as "the theory that parts of a whole are in intimate connection, such that they cannot exist independently of the whole or cannot be understood without reference to the whole, which is thus greater than the sum of its parts" (Wikipedia 2020 para 1). Holistic management denotes the ability of those who manage organizations to see organizations not only as one whole but also to have the ability to create infrastructures that truly connect all parts of the organization to produce the whole. The concept of reductionism within the context of holism was discussed in chapter 2, reflecting the nature of nursing home operation where there too many parts of the system that need to be connected to form a whole.

Nursing homes are no longer admitting residents needing only custodial care. Current residents in nursing homes are sicker, most with multi-morbidities and therefore candidates for potential or frequent unplanned hospitalization. In an article titled "Medicare Take Aim at Boomerang Hospitalization of Nursing Home Patients," Rau (2018) wrote that "with hospitals pushing patients out of there earlier, nursing homes are deluged with increasingly frail patients . . . with their sometimes skeletal medical staffing, often fail to handle post-hospital complications" (Wikipedia, 2020, para 6). In the face of these new realities in nursing home care, there is a need for those who manage or own nursing homes to rethink how to embrace holistic management principles as a lifelong activity to enable them to address the public demand for change and to remain in compliance with nursing home care regulatory requirements.

To achieve nursing home quality, there is a need for regulators, administrators, and care providers to reflect on a few main items that require additional review for improvement. There is need for an in-depth understanding of the implications of the two main systems that exist interdependently in nursing homes—the holistic resident care management, a.k.a. resident-centered care, and the holistic nursing home business management; understanding of the impact nursing staffing shortages/workload/low wages for CNAs has on residents' quality and quantity of care; understanding of the impact the frontline staff supervision has on residents' quality and quantity of care; understanding of the impact of a single-room dwelling versus room-mating has on residents' need for privacy, independence, and control; understanding of the complexities of nursing home caregiving beyond what it presents on the surface; understanding of the psychosocial impact of a nursing home being a 24/7 workplace for staff as well as a home for the residents; understanding the impact of overtime on resident quality of care; and understanding of the need for integration of all parts of the nursing home systems into one whole.

Finally, it is our observation that the issues listed herein are sociomanagement issues, with their impact of undermining clinical/medical performance in nursing homes. The problem of poor nursing home quality does not lie in more government regulation—unless absolutely necessary—but in the lack of holistic approach to management, for which the entrepreneurial owners of nursing homes are responsible.

In the past, and despite OBRA's definition of the term "comprehensive," nursing home operation was still viewed almost exclusively from the clinical/

medical perspective. Nursing home residents may have wounds that need treatment or medications to treat or control disease process, but in holistic nursing home management, resident needs are multidimensional, with each need having an absolute value to the resident that must not be neglected.

Administrators' Daily Quiz

In a holistic nursing home management, which of the following objective is the most important to you and your organization?

A. Maintain the highest resident's quality care
B. Maintain the highest daily census
C. Maintain the highest staffing and staff motivational levels
D. A & B
E. A & C
F. B & C
G. None of the above
H. All of the above

References

Alimohammadlou, M., and Eslamloo, F. "Relationship Between Total Quality Management, Knowledge Transfer and Knowledge Diffusion in the Academic Settings." *Procedia*, 230 (2016), 104–111.doi: 10.1016/j.sbspro.2016.09.013 "Almshouse Care," 2. (2004, March 10). *Almshouse Care*. Retrieved from Maryland State Archives: Retrieved from http://msa.maryland.gov/msa/speccol/sc5400/sc5492/html/almshouse_ii.htm

Al-Shdaifat, E. A. "Implementation of Total Quality Management in Hospitals." *Journal of Taibah University Medical Sciences*, 10(4), 461–466 (2015): https://doi.org/10.1016/j.jtumed.2015.05.004

Allen, Marshall. "One-Third of Skilled Nursing Patients Harmed in Treatment." Retrieved from propublica.org/article/one-third-of-skilled-nursing-patients-harmed-in-treatment (2014).

Amagoh, Francis. "Leadership Development and Leadership Effectiveness." Retrieved from emerald.com/insight/content/doi/10.1110 8/00251740910966695/full/html (2011).

Anderson, Jane. "Study finds Oldest Old Are Shifting from NHs. Caring for Ages: A Monthly Newspaper for Long Term Practitioners," January 2007, Vol., No. 1, p.12.

Anderson, Ruth A. Issel, Michele L., and McDaniel, Reuben R. "Nursing Homes as Complex Adaptive Systems: Relationship between Management

Practice and Resident Outcomes." Retrieved from https://www.ncbi.nlm.nih.gov/pmc/articles/PMC1993902/ (2007).

Ayanian, J. Z. and Markel H. "Donabedian's Lasting Framework for Health Care Quality." Retrieved from hcp.med.harvard.edu/publications/donabedian's-lasting-framework-health-care-quality (2016).

Babalola et al(2014). "Building a Health Information Technology Infrastructure in Long-Term Care." Retrieved from semanticscholar.org/paper/Building-a-Health-Information-Technology-in-Care-Babalola-Bair/4b22dOe59826d5fb7ec3cc76f17f3fe79bb7df51.

Berwick, Donald and Fox Daniel M. "Evaluating the Quality of Medical Care": Donabedian's Classic Article 50 Years Later. Retrieved from ncbi.nlm.nih.gov/PMC/articles/PMC4911723/ (2016).

Benner, Carol. "It's All about Change." Delmarva Foundation Presentation, May 24, 2006. p. 10.

Bethel, Sheila Murray. *Making a Difference: 12 Qualities that Make You a Leader* (New York, The Berkley Publishing Group: 1990.

Bailey, Diana. "Budgeting for Employee Engagement. Retrieved from honestly.com/blog/budgeting-employee-engagement/ (2018).

Blanchard, Sarah. 6 Signs of Nursing Home Neglect. Retrieved from htt://www.nextavenue.org/6-signs-of-nursing-home-neglect/ (2016).

Blanchard, Kenneth and Johnson Spencer. *The One Minute Manager.* (New York, The Berkerley Publishing Group, 1982).

Bloch, H. "Medicine and Science in the 19th and 20th Centuries." *Journal of the National dical Association*, 229–232.

Bloomenthal, Andrew. "Organizational Chart." Retrieved from investopedia.com/teams/o/organizational-chart.asp (2019).

Bolton, Robert and Dorothy Grover Bolton. *Social Style/ Management Style: Developing Productive Work Relationships* (New York, American Management Associations, Publication Group: 1984).

Bormann, Ernest G et al. *Interpersonal Communication in the Modern Organization* (Englewood Cliff, New Jersey, Prentice-Hall, Inc.: 1969).

Bradford, Alina. "What is a Theory?" Retrieved from livescience. com/21491-what-is-a-scientific-theory-definition-of-theory.html (2017).

Brown, Douglas J. *The Human Nature of Organizations* (New York, AMACOM, 1973).

Brown, Reva Berman and Sean McCartney. "A Home from Home: The Organization as Family." Retrieved from tandfonline.com/doi/abs/10.1080/10245289608523478? (2017).

Burke, Steven S. and Tessa L. Chenaille."30 Essential Policies and Procedures for Long-Term Care." Retrieved from hcmarketplace.com/media/supplemental/3856-browse.pdf (2006).

Buttigieg, S., P. K. Dey and D. Gauci. "Business Process Management in Healthcare: Current Challenges and Future Prospects." *Innovation and Entrepreneurship in Health*: 3, 11–13. https://doi.org/10.2147/IEH. S68183 (2015).

Carleton, W. *Farm Ballads* (New York: Harper and Collins, 1882).

Castle, P. M. "What is Nursing Home Quality and How is It Measured?" *The Gerontologist* (2010): 426–442.

Cherry, Kendra. "The Situational Theory of Leadership." Retrieved from verywellmind.com/what-is-the-situational-theory-of-leadership-279321 (2019).

CMS.gov. "QAPI Description and Background." Retrieved from https://www.cms.gov/medicare/provider-enrollment-and-certification/QAPI/qapidefinition.html (2016).

Cofer, C.N. and M/ H. Appley. *Motivation: Theory and Research* (New York: John Wiley and Sons, Inc.

Cole, Nicolas (2017). "3 Critical Reasons Employees Become Unmotivated In The Workplace." Retrieved from inc.com/nicolas-cole/3-critical-reasons-employees-become-unmotivated-in-the-workplace.html

Coleman, James C. *Abnormal Psychology and Modern Life* (Illinois, Scott Foresman and Company, 1972).

Corbet, Barry. Embedded, AARP. *The Magazine*, January–February (2007), p. 54.

Covey, Stephen R. *The 7 Habits of Highly Effective People* (New York, Simon & Schuster, 1989).

Cox, Harold. *Aging* (Guilford, Connecticut: The Dushkin Publishing Group, Inc., 1989).

Crannell, L. *Historical Overview of the American Poorhouse System*. Retrieved from The Poor House Story : Retrieved from http://www.poorhousestory.com/history.htm (2000).

Dana, Bernie and Olson Dauglas (nd). "Effective Leadership in Long Term Care: The Need and the Opportunity." Retrieved from achca.memberclick.net/assets/docs/AHCA-Leadership-Need-and-Opportunity-Paper-Dana-Olson-pdf

Darson, Sandy. Traditional Nursing Vs .Holistic Nursing. Retrieved from www.healthcare.com/articles/view.php?article-id=13769 (2013).

Derlega, Valerian J. and Louis H. Janda. *Personal Adjustment: The Psychology of Everyday Life, Second Edition* (Glenview, Illinois: Scott Foresman and Company, 1981).

Dewitt, Anthony L. "When Falls Mean Negligence, Advance for Long Term Care Management," May–June 2007, p.24.

Dickson, John. "Nursing Home Quality: Continued Improvements Needed in CMS's Data and Oversight." Retrieved from https://www.gao.gov/products/GAO-18-694T (2018).

Dock, Lavinia. "Almshouse Nursing." *The American Journal of Nursing* (1908): 361–363.

Doddi, Srikar. "Three Approaches to Deal with Bounded Rationality." Retrieved from https://medium.com/pminsider/three-approaches-to-deal-with-bounded-rationality-dde5cd7d5ce2 (2018).

Donabedian, A. "The Seven Pillars of Quality." Retrieved from pubmed.ncbi.nlm.nih.gov/2241519/ (1990).

Drucker, Peter F. *Management Tasks Responsibilities Practices* (Toronto, Fitzhenry & Whiteside Limited: 1973).

Dubin, Robert. A Theory of Conflict and Power in Union-Management Relations. Retrieved from jstor.org/stable/2520201?=1 (1960).

Ellerman, Lauren. "Why Nursing Home Policies and Procedures Are so Important." Retrieved from https://frithlawfirm.com/blog/medical/nursing-homes/why-nursing-home-policies-and-procedures-are-so-important/ (2016).

Ersek, Mary. Transforming Nursing Home Care. Retrieved from https://opinionator.blogs.nytimes.com/2015/04/01/transforming-nursing-home-care/

Fabry, Joseph B (1968). The Pursuit of Meaning, Cork and Dublin, The Mercier Press (2015).

Felder, Robin. "Medical Automation—A Technologically Enhanced Work Environment to Reduce the Burden of Care on Nursing Staff and a Solution to the Care Cost Crises." *Nursing Outlook*. (May/June 2003): p. S7.

Flanagan, Nina. "QAPI: Nursing Challenges and Successes." Retrieved from https://www.caringfortheages.com/article/S1526-4114(17)30095-1/pdf (2017).

Fleek, Carole. "Double Blind," *AARP Bulletin*, Vol. 47, No. 5 (2006): p. 18.

Forbes, Sharine. *Why Do Seniors Often Resist Living in a Nursing Home*. Retrieved from sharecare.com/user/sharine?currentPage=2 (2012).

Foroux, Darius." On the Cyclical Nature of Life". Retrieved from dariusforoux.com/cyclical-nature-of-life/ (2020).

Fromm, Eric. *To Have or To Be: World Perspectives*, Volume 50 (New York, Harper & Row Publishers, 1976).

Funk, Jim. "9 Characteristics of Holistic Leaders." Retrieved from eocnam.org/2016/07/15/9-characteristics-of-holistic-leaders/ (2016).

Galinato, Jose, Mary Montie, Lance Patak, Titler. "Perspective of Nurses and Patients on Call Light Technology." Retrieved from https://www.ncbi.nim.nih.gov/pmc/articles/PMC4546527/ (2016).

Ghose, Tia. "Just a Theory: 7 Misused Science Words." Retrieved from scientificamerican.com/article/just-a-theory-7-misused-science-words/ (2013).

Ghoshal, Sumantra (n d). "Bad Management Theories Are Destroying Good Management Practices." Retrieved from C:/User/Owner/Downloads/BadManagementtheoriesVsGoodmanagementpractices%20(2).pdf

Goldebert, Amy and Kathleen Shostek. "Creating a Culter of Safety, ECPN: Clinical and Financial Strategies for the Extended Care Professional." (April 2007): p. 18–20.

Goldsmith, Seth B. *Long-Term Care Administration Handbook* (Gaithersburg, Maryland, Aspen Publishers, Inc.): 1993.

Gordon, George Kenneth and Stryker Ruth. *Creative Long-Term Care Administration.* (Charles C. Thomas, Illinois, 1983).

Gourevitch, M. W. "The Public Hospital in American Medical Education." *Journal of Urban Health* (2008) 779–786.

Greenberg, Barry." Nursing Home Facilities and Housekeeping: Odor and Stain Control." Retrieved from chemeindustries.com/blog/nursing-facilities-and-housekeeping-odor-and-stain-control (2016).

Grensing-Pophal, Lin. "Uncovering 2 Types of Authority." Retrieved from hrdailyadvisor.blr.com/2019/05/06/uncovering-2-types-of-authority/ (2019).

Gruneir, Andrea and Vincent Mor. "Nursing Home Safety: Current Issues and Barriers to Imorvement." Retrieved from pubed.ncbi.nil.nih.gov/18173385 (2008).

Harkins, Malcolm J. "The Broken Promise of OBRA '87: The Failure to Validate the Survey Protocol." Retrieved from slu.edu/law/academics/journals/health-law-policy/pdf/issues/v8-i1/harkins-article-1.pdf (2014).

Harrington, Charlene et al. "Appropriate Nursing Staffing Levels for US Nursing Homes." Retrieved from journals.sagepub.com/doi/full/10.1177/1178632920934785 (2020).

Harris-Wehling, Jo. "Defining Quality of Care." Retrieved from https://www.ncbi.nli.gov/books/NBK235476/ (1990).

Havig, Anders Kvale et al. "Leadsership, Staffing and Quality of Care in Nursing Homes." Retrieved from ncbi.nlm.nih.gov/books/NBK232673/ (2011).

Hawes, Catherine and Charles D. "The Changing Structure of the Nursing Home Industry and the Impact of Ownership on Quality, Cost, and Access." Retrieved from https://www.ncbi.nlh.gov/books/NBK217907/ (1986).

Hernandez, Lauren. "Thomas More: What Is the Ideal Society?: Retrieved from https://prezi.com/jzixrfloutov/thomas-more-what-is-the-ideal-society/ Number 2, p. 26 (2015).

Hersey, Paul, Kenneth H. Blanchard, Dewet E. Johnson. *Management of Organizational Behavior: Leading Human Resources*. (New Jersey, Prentice-Hall Inc., Eight Edition, 2001).

Heshmat, Shahram. "Satisficing Vs Maximizing." Retrieved from psychologytoday.com/us/blog/science-choice/201506/satisficing-vs-maximizing (2015).

Holland, Michael." What Is Leadership Style and Why Does it Matter to Me." Retrieved from bishophouse.com/your-development/why-your-should-understand-your-leadership-style/ (2017).

Hooyman, Nancy R. and Asuman H. Kiyak. *Social Gerontology: A Multidisciplinary Perspective*. (Boston. Allyn and Bacon, Inc., 1988).

Horn, L., and E. Griesel. *Nursing Homes: A Citizen's Action Guide* (Boston: Beacon Press, 1977).

Husain, Zareen. "Effective Communication Brings Successful Organizational Change." Retrieved from https://www.abrmr.com/myfile/conference-proceedings/con-Pro-12315/7-dubai13 (2013).

Jacobson, Greg. "5 Principles of a High Reliability Organization." Retrieved from blog.kainexus.com/improvement-disciplines/hro/5-principles (2019).

Jenney, Kelli. "The Contempt of the Poor: A Closer Look into New York City Almshouses in the Nineteenth-Century and the Treatment of the Lower Class." Retrieved from digitalcommons.providence.edu/cgi/viewcontent.cgi?article=1001&context=history-undergrad-thesis (2019).

Johannsen, F. "A holistic Approach for Integrating Methods in Quality Management." Retrieved from http://www.wi2013.de/proceedings/WI2013%20-%20Track%206%20-%20Johannsen.pdf (2013).

Kaktins, M. *The Encyclopedia of Greater Philadelphia.* Retrieved from Philadelphia Encyclopedia: http://philadelphiaencyclopedia.org/archive/almshouses-poorhouses/ (2016).

Kapp, M. B. "At least Mom Will Be Safe There: The Role of Resident safety in Nursing Home Quality." Retrieved from https//www.ncbi.nlh.gov/pmc/articles/PMC1743720/ (2003).

Kaykas-wolff, Jascha. "Incentive Vs. Motivation." Retrieved from medium.com/agile-marketing/incentive-vs-motivation-51adb8c04cef (2015).

Kessler, E. J. (Ed.). *Encyclopedia of Management Theory* (Thousand Oaks, California: Sage Publications, 2013). Retrieved from http://www.gervasebushe.ca/the_AI_model.pdf

Kheirandish, Reza and Shabnam Mousavi. "Herbert Simon, Innovation, and Heuristics." Retrieved from link.spinger.com/article/10.1007/s11299-019-00203-6 (2019).

Kluwer, Wolter. "What Are QAPI Programs in Long-Term Care?" Retrieved from Lipincottsolution.lww.com/blog.entry.html/2017/11/27/what-are-qapi-progra-tfxO.html (2017).

Kneller, George F. Editor. *Foundations of Education*, Third Edition (New York, John Wiley and Sons, 1976).

Knickman, James R. and Emily K. Snell. "The 2030 Problem: Caring for Aging Baby Boomers." Retrieved from ncbi.nlm.nih.gov/pmc/articles/PMC1464018/ (2002).

Konetzka, Tamara. "The Challenges of Improving Nursing Home Quality." Retriewed from jamanetwork.com/journals/jamanetworkopen/fullarticle/2759755 (2020).

Kokemuller, Neil. "The Difference Between Leadership & Supervising." Retrieved from smallbusiness.chron.com/difference-between-leadership-supervising-42168.html (2020).

Kuehner-Herbert, Katie. "The Importance of Holistic Approach to Employee Management." Retrieved from https://www benefitspro.com/2018/08/14/the-importance-of-a-holistic-approach-to-employee/ (2018)

Larcher, Bob. "Holistic Leadership." Retrieved from boblarcher.com/Holistic.pdf (2020).

Larson, Dana. "The Green House Project: The Next Big Thing in Long-Term Care." Retrieved from aplaceformom.com/caregiver-resources/articles/green-house-project-long-term-care (2015).

Lawal, A. K., T. Rotter, L. Kinsman, N. Sari, L. Harrison, C. Jeffery, R. Flynn. "Lean Management in Healthcare: Definition, Concepts, Methodology and Effects Reported (systematic review protocol). *Systematic Reviews*, 3, 103.doi: 10.1186/2046-4053-3-103 (2014).

Learning, Elite. "Nursing Overtime: The Good, The Bad, The OMG." Retrieved from elitecme.com/resource-center/nursing/nursing-overtime-the-good-the bad-the omg (2018).

Leatherbarrow, Jennifer. "QAPI Basics—The Five Elements and 12 Steps." Retrieved from http://blog.richterc.com/qapi-basics-the-five-elemenrs-and-twelve-steps (2016).

Lenzer, Jeanne. "The Future of Healthcare Is Here: The Pandemic Has Turned Telehealth from a May One Day to a Right Here, Right Now." *AARP Bulletin* (June 2020): vol. 61, no. 5.

Levene, Abbey. "What is the Right Organizational Structure for the 21st Century." Retrieved from blog.dropbox.com/topics/work-culture/21st-century-organization-structure (2020).

Li, Yue and Cai. "Racial and Ethnic Disparities in Social Engahement among US Nursing Home Residents." Retrieved from ncbi.nlm.nih.gov/pmc/articles/PMC4031618/ (2014).

Liebert, Robert M., and Michael D. Spiegler. *Personality: Strategies for the Study of Man, Revised Version* (Illinois: The Dorsey Homewood, 1974).

Light, Kathleen M. "Florence Nightingale and Holistic Philosophy." Retrieved from https://www.ncbi.nih.gov/pubmed/9146193.

Litka, Michael P. and James E. Inman. *The Legal Environment of Business: Text, Cases and Readings* (Columbus, Ohio: Grid, Inc., 1975).

Lykins, Alexander. "The Business Case for 'Holistic Management.'" Retrieved from greenbiz.com/article/business-case-holistic-management (2017).

Madlinger, Grace. "73 Employee Engagement Ideas for Any Budget." Retrieved from wheniwork.com/blog.73/09/73-employee-engagement-ideas-for-any-budget (2019).

McCormick, Ernest J., and Joseph Tiffin. *Industrial Psychology, Sixth Edition* (Englewood Cliffs).

McCroskey, Richmond and McCroskey. "The Nature of Communication in Organization." Retrieved from my.ilstu/~llipper/com329/mccroskey-chapter.pdf (2005).

McCullough, Laurence B. and Nancy L. Wilson. *Long-Term Care Decisions Ethical and Conceptual Dimensions* (Baltimore: The Johns Hopkins University Press, 1995).

McPherson, Judith R. "Program Manager's Memo to Administrator on Complains or Unusual Incident in Nursing Facilities," Government of the District of Columbia, Department of health, Licensing Regulation Administration, 2000, 614 H Street, Rm. 1003, Washington, DC 2000, p.1

Meibner, Anne and Wilfred Schnepp. "Staff Experiences within the Implementation of Computer-Based Nursing Records in Residential Aged Care Facilities: A Systematic Review and Synthesis Of Qualitative Research." Retrieved from https://bmcmedinformdecismak.biomedcentral.com/articles/10.1186/1472-6947-14-54 (2014).

Menio et al. "The Nursing Staffing in Nursing Homes." Retrieved from theconsumervoice.org/uploads/files/issues/Consensus-Statement-Staffing.pdf (2001).

Merrill, Francis E. *Society and Culture: An Introduction to Sociology. Fourth Edition* (Englewood Cliff, New Jersey: Prentice-Hall, Inc., 1969).

Miller, Harry L. *Teaching and Learning in Adult Education* (New York: The Macmillan Company, 1964).

Millett, John D. *Organization for the Public Service* (New York: D. VAN NOSTRAND Company, Inc., 1966)

Moore, K. L., W. J. Boscardin, M. A. Steinman, J. B. and Schwartz. "Patterns of Chronic Co-morbid Medical Conditions in Older Residents of U.S. Nursing Homes: Differences between the Sexes and Across Age-Span." Retrieved from https://www.nibi.nlm.nih.gov/pmc/articles/PMC4099251/ (2018).

Moorer, K., S. Kunupakaphun, E. Delgado, M. Moody, C. Wolf, K. Moore, and P. Eamranond. "Using Appreciative Inquiry as a Framework to Enhance the Patient Experience." *Patient Experience Journal*, 4(3). 8

Morford, Thomas G. "Nursing Home Regulation: History and Expectations." Retrieved from https://www.ncbi.nlm.nib.gov/pmc/articles/PMC4195121/ (1988).

Morgan, Jacob. "Why the Millions We Spend On Employee Engagement Buy Us So Little." Retrieved from hbr.org/2017/03/why-the-millions-we-spend-on-employee- engagement-buy-us-so-little (2017).

Mosadeghrad, A. M. "Toward a Theory of Quality Management: An Integration of Strategic Management, Quality Management and Project Management." *International Journal of Modeling of Operations Management*, 2(1) (2012): 89–118.do.:

Mousa, A. "Lean, Six Sigma, and Lean Six Sigma Overview." *International Journal of Scientific & Engineering Research*, 4(5) (2013) 1137–1153.

Nappi, Rebecca. "The Spokesman-Review." Retrieved from www.spokesman.com/stories/2012/apr/15/when-it-comes-to-trying-to-rename-that-infamous/ (2012).

Nochomovitz, Emma (n.d.). "Skilled Nursing Facilities and Other Long Term Care Facilities Addressing Issues of Cost and Quality." Retrieved from http://www.cwru.edu/med/epidbio/mphp439/nursing_homes.pdf

Northouse, Peter G. *Leadership: Theory and Practice* (United Kindom, Sage Publications, Inc., 2013).

"Nursing Homes and Assisted Living (Long-Term Facilities [LTCFs])." (Centers for Disease Control, 2017). Retrieved from https://www.cdc.gov/longtermcare/

O'connell, Brian (2019). What Is Opportunity Cost and What Does It Mean for You. Retrieved from https://www.thestreet.com/personal-finance/opportunity-cost-14648358

O' Connor, John. "Don't Forget Why You're Here, McKnight's Long Term Care News" (January: 18).Olds, M., Danielle and Sean P. Clarke. "The Effect of Work Hours on Adverse Event and Errors In Health Care." Retrieved from ncbi.nlm.nih.gov/pmc/articles.PMC2910393/ (2011).

Omare, Osamudiamen Kelvin. "7 Ways Parents Work to Destroy Their Child's Future Success." Retrieved from thriveglobal.com/stories/7-ways-parents-work-to-destroy-their-child-s-future/ (2017).

Pate, Terri and Stacy Yale. *The Facility Guide to OBRA Regulations and the Long-Term Care Survey Process* (Miamisburg, Ohio: 45342, MED-PASS, Inc., 2017).

Pate, Terri and Staup Yale. *The Facility Guide to OBRA Regulations, and the Long Term Care Survey Process, 2005 Edition* (MEDPASS, Inc., 2005).

Pennington et al. "The Role of Certified Nursing Assistants in Nuring Homes." Retrieved from nursingcenter.com/journalarticle?Article-ID=429063&journal-ID54024&Issues-ID429045 (2003).

Poels, Joris et al. "Leadership Styles and Leadership Outcomes in Nursing Homes: A Cross-Sectional Analysis." Retrieved from bmchealthservres. biomedcentral.com/articles/10.1186/s12913-020-05854-7 (2020).

Porvaznik, Jan. "The Concept of the Holistic Management as a New Approach in the Theory of Management." Retrieved from https://mpra. ub.uni-muenchen.de/57444/1/MPRA-paper-57444.pdf (2014).

Powillis, S., Ed. "Residents Say Quality of Life is lacking in Long Term Care Setting." *McKnight's Long Term Care News* (1990): 12–20.

Quain, Sampson. "Positive & Negative Effects of Employee Motivation." Retrieved from smallbusiness.chron.com/positive-negative-effects-employee-motivation-14535.html (2019).

Rabin, David L. and Patricia Stockton. *Long-Term Care Fort the Elderly: A Fact Book* (New York, Oxford University Press, 1987).

Rakich, Johnathan S., Beaufort B. Longest, Kurt Darr. *Managing Healthy Services Organizations, Second Edition* (Philadelphia, W.B. Saunders Company, 1977).

Rau, Jordan. "Medicaid Takes Aim at Boomerang Hospitalizations of Nursing Home Patients." Retrieved from khn.org/news/medicare-takes-aim-at-boomerang-hospitalizatios-of-nursing-home-patients/ (2018).

Reimers, David M. "Post-World War II Immigration to the United States: America's Latest Newcomers" Retrieved from journals.sagepub.com/doi/abs/10.1177/000271628145400102 (1981).

Reynolds, Paddy (n d). "Holistic Management—Inside-outside Management." Retrieved from insideoutsidemgt.com.au/holistic-management.

Rhoades, Jefferey A. *The Nursing Home Market: Supply and Demand for the Elderly* (New York and London, Garland Publishing, Inc., 1998).

Riggio, Ronald. "Leaders: Born or Made." Retrieved from psychology.com/us/blog/cutting-edge-leadership/200903/leaders-born-or-made (2020).

Rosen, Jule. "Administering Venlafaxine in Nursing Homes. When do the Benefits Outweigh theRisk," *Long Term Care Interface*, Vol. 8 (March–April 2007): Regulation Administration, Washington, DC, p. 31.

Rubertino, Frosini. "Quality Assurance and Performance Improvement: A nursing Home Guide to Implementation and Management." Retrieved from https://hcmarketplace.com/aitdownloadablefiles/download/aitfile/aitfile-id/1570.pdf (2014).

Rust, Betsy. "Nursing Homes Fade Even as Baby Boomers Age." Retrieved from https://www.statnews.com/2016/06/23/nursing-homes-fade-baby-boomers-age/ (2016).

Saunders, Elizabeth Grace. "A Holistic Approach to Business." Retrieved from sbnonline.com/article/a-holistic-approach-to-business-how-broad-business-knowledge-help-employees-thrive/ (2007).

Sfantou, D. F., A. Laliotis, E. Patelarou, D. Sifaki-Pistolla, M. Matalliotakis, and E. Patelarou. "Importance of Leadership Style Toward Quality of Care Measures in Healthcare Settings: A Systematic Review." Retrieved from pubmed.ncbi.nlm.nih.gov/29036901/ (2017).

Siberski, James and Carol Siberski (n .d). "Boomers in Nursing Homes: Ready or Not, Here They Come." Retrieved from todaysgeriatricmedicine. com/archieve/0915p18.shtml.

Siddiqui, Fareed. "The Importance of Behavioral Science in Business Management." Retrieved from https://www.Linkin.com/pulse/importance-behavioral-science-business-management-fareed (2015).

Siegel, E. O. and L. Zysberg. "Licensed Nursing Home Administrator Preparation and Role Variations," *Annals of Long-Term Care: Clinical Care and Aging*, 24(3) (2016): 28–36.

Simwanza, Limichilwe. "On the Cyclical Nature of Life." Retrieved from medium.com/the-post-grad-survival-guide/on-the-cyclical-nature-of-life-9450294bd117 (2018).

Smikle, Joanne. "The Pivotal Role of the Nursing Home Administrator Provider." Retrieved from http://www.providermagazine.com/ archives/2014_Archives/Pages/0814/The-Pivotal-Role-Of-The-Nursing-Home-Administrator.aspx (2014).

Smith, Karl and William M. Smith. *The Behavior of Man: Introduction of Psychology* (University of Wisconsin, Henry Holt and Company, Inc., 1958).

Solis, Brian. "The Time Has Come for Holistic Business Strategy." Retrieved from fastcompany.com/1719518/time-has-come-holistic-business-strategy (2011).

Surbhi, S. "Difference Between Power and Authority." Retrieved from keydifferences.com/difference-between-power-and-authority.html (2016).

Strauss, Valerie. "What's the Purpose of Education in the 21st Century?" Retrieved from washingtonpost.com/news/answer-sheet/wp/2015/02/12/ what's-the-purpose-of-education-in-the-21st-century/ (1915).

Teich, S. T., and F. F. Faddoul. "Lean management—The Journey from Toyota to Healthcare," *Rambam Maimonides Medical Journal*, 4(2), e0007. doi:10.5041/RMMJ.10107 (2013).

Terrace, Bryn Mawr. "How Effective Communication with Long-Term Care Staff Achieves the Best Care." Retrieved from brynmawrterrace.org/article/12/22/2015/how-effective-communication-long-term-care-staff-achieves-best-care (2015).

Tzeng, Huey-Ming. "Perspectives of Patients and Families about the Nature of and Reasons for Call Light Use and Staff Call Light ResponseTime," *Medsurg Nursing*, Volume 20, No. 5 (2011): 225.

Umoren, Joseph A. *A Study of Factors Related to the Educational Decisions and Career Plans of Secondary School Seniors in One Nigerian State to Pursue or Not to Pursue Higher Education* (University Microfilms International, A bell and Howell Information Company, 1989).

Umoren, Joseph A. "Maslow's Hierarchy of Needs and OBRA 1987: Toward Need Satisfaction by Nursing Home Resident's Educational Gerontology: An International Journey," Vol., 18, Number 6, (September 1992): 665.

Van den Brink, Anne M. A., Debby L. Gerritsen, Richard C. Oude Voshaar, and Raymond T. C. Koopmans. "Resident with Mental-Physical Multi-morbidity Living in Long-Term Care Facilities: Prevalence and Characteristics. A Systematic Review." Retrieved from https://www.cambridge.org/core/journals/international-psychogeriatrics/article/residents-with-mentalphysical-multimorbidity-living-in-longterm-care-facilities-prevalence-and-characteristics-a-systematic-view/0A4B4FDDAA91B9570D5A4398B288AABA (2012).

Wagner, D. "The Poorhouse: America's Forgotten Institution." Retrieved from The Social Welfare Library VCU: Retrieved from http://socialwelfare.library.vcu.edu/issues/poor-relief-almshouse/ (2005).

Walshe, Kieran. "Regulating U.S. Nursing Homes: Are We Learning From Experience?" Retrieved from https://doi.org/10.1377/hlthaff.20.6.128 (2001).

Wiener, Joshua M. "An Assessment of Strategies for Improving Quality of Care in Nursing Homes." Retrieved from academic.coup.com/gerontologist/ article/43/suppl-2/19/637521 (2003).

Wilkins, Alasdair. "How a Pair of Astrologers Helped Invent Modern Medical Record-Keeping." Retrieved from https://io9.gizimodo.com/how-a-pair-of-astrologers-helped-invent-modern-medical-5850286 (2011).

Yasir Muhammad, Iman Rabia, Irshad Muhammad Kashif, Mohamad Noor Azmi, Khan Muhammad Muddassar. "Leadership Styles in Relation to Employees' Trust and Organizational Change Capacity: Evidence From Non-profit Organizations." Retrieved from journals.sagepub.com/doi/ pdf/10.1177/2158244016675396 (2015).

Zamanzadeh, V., M. Jasemi, L. Valizadeh, B. Keogh, and F. Taleghani. "Effective Factors in Providing HolisticCare: A Qualitative Study," *Indian Journal of Palliative Care*, 21(2), 214-224.doi:10.4103/0973-1075.156506 (2015).

———. "Update on the Public Views of Nursing Homes and Long-Term Care Services." Retrieved from https://www.kff.org/other/poll-finding/ update-on-the-public-views-of-nursing/ (2007).

———. *Webster's 11 New Riverside Dictionary* (Boston, Houghton Muffin Company, 1996).

——— . *District of Columbia Municipal Regulations (DCMR)* (Department of Health, Health, Health, 2001).

———. "Fraud and Abuse Watch," *Long Term Care Interface*, Volume 7, Number 1 (January 2006): 42.

————. *Facility Guide to OBRA Regulations, Interpretive Guidelines and the LTC Survey Process, 2001 Edition* (Heaton Resources, MEDPASS, Inc., 2001).

Wikipedia. "Almshouse." Retrieved from https://en.wikipedia.org/wiki/Almshouse

Wikipedia. "American Holistic Medical Association." Retrieved from faim.org/american-holistic-medical-association-ahma

Wikipedia. "Baby Boomer Trends." Retrieved from https://nabbw.com/free-resources/baby-boomer-trends/

Wikipedia. "Baby Boomers Will Become Sicker Seniors than Earlier generations." Retrieved from www.npt.org/sections/health-shots/2016/05/25/479359856/baby-boomers-will-become sicker-seniors- than-earlier-generations

Wikipedia. "Baby Boomers Will Transform Health Care as They Age." Retrieved from www.hhnmag.com/articles/5298-Boomers-will-Transform-Health-Care-as-They-Age

Wikipedia. "Boomers in Nursing Homes: Ready or Not, Here They Come." Retrieved from www.todaysgeriatricsmedicine.com/archieve/0915p18.shtml

Wikipedia. "Crosswalk-Old and New Federal Nursing Home Regulations." Retrieved from dhs.wisconsin.gov/publications/p)1943.pdf

Wikipedia. "David Brownstein." Retrieved from https//:www.alibris.com/search/books/author/David-Brownstein

Wikipedia. "Effective Supervision." Retrieved from www.3nd.edu/-jthomp19/2-spring%20semester/effective-supervision-v2.pdf

Wikipedia. "Holistic Industries Overview." Retrieved from glassdoor.com/overview/Working-at-Holistic-Industies-EI-IE2475229.11,30.htm

Wikipedia. "Nightingale's Environmental Theory." Retrieved from https://en.wikipedia.org/wiki/Nightingale%27s-environmental/-theory

Wikipedia. *"Using Change Concepts for Improvement."* Retrieved from www.ihi.org/resources/Pages/Changes/UsingChangeConceptsforImprovement.aspx

Wikipedia. "Bloom's Taxonomy." Retrieved from https://en.wikipedia.org/wiki/Bloom%27s-taxonomy

Wikipedia. "Chronic Diseases and Health Promotion: Integrated Chronic Disease Prevention and Control." Retrieved from www.who.int/chp/about/integrated -cd/en/

Wikipedia. "Comorbidity." Retrieved from https://.wikipedia.org/wiki/Comorbidity

Wikipedia. "Federal Requirements of Participation for Nursing Homes Issued September 2016 Summary of Key Changes in the Rule-Part 2." Retrieved from theconsumervoice.org/uploads/files/issues/summry-of-key-changes-effective-phase-1-part2-final pdf

Wikipedia. "Admissions Policy." Retrieved from licamedman.com/ftag/596/f620-admissions-policy

Wikipedia. "IOM Definition of Quality." Retrieved from https://www.google.com/search?q=iom+definition+of+quality&oq=IOM+definition+of+&aqs=chrome.0.0j69i57j0l4.42062j1j8&sourceid=chrome&ie=UTF-8

Wikipedia. "Incentive and Motivation—What's the difference?" Retrieved from incentiveandmotivation.com/incentive-motivation-whats-the-difference

Wikipedia. "John Dewey." Retrieved from https://www.google.com/search?q=john+dewey+theory&oq=john+Dewey&aqs=chrme.2.69i59j0l5.134

Wikipedia. "Medical Conditions of Nursing Home Admissions." Retrieved from https://bmcgeriatr.biomedcentral.com/articles/10.1186/1471-2318-10-46

Wikipedia. "Nursing Homes and Assisted Living (Long-term Care Facilities [LTCFs]." Retrieved from https://www.cdc.gov/longtermcare/index.html

Wikipedia. "Satisficing." Retrieved from https://en.wikipedia.org/wiki/Satisficing

Wikipedia. "Understanding the Social Psychology of Risk and Safety." Retrieved from https://safetyrisk.net/understanding-the-social-psychology-of-risk-and-safety/

Wikipedia. "Chester Bernard." Retrieved from https://en.wikipedia.org/wiki/Chester-Bernard

Wikipedia. "Constitutional Law." Retrieved from https://en.wikipedia.org/wiki/constitutional law.

Wikipedia. "Contingency Theory." Retrieved from en.wikipedia/wiki/contingency-theory

Wikipedia. "Policy." Retrieved from https://en.m.wikipedia.org/wiki/policy

Wikipedia. "What Is Leadership?" Retrieved from https://www.mindtools.com/pages/article/newLDR-41.htm

Wikipedia. "Long-Term Care in the United States: A Timeline." Retrieved from Kff.org/Medicaid/timeline/long-term-care-in-the-United States-a-timeline/

Wikipedia. "Henri Fayol's Principles of Management: Early Management Theory." Retrieved from mindtools.com/pages/articles/henri-fayol.htm

Wikipedia. "The Industrial Revolution and Its Impact on Family Life and Women." Retrieved from https://www.bartleby.com/essay/The-Industrial Revolution-and-Its-Impact-on-F3CN7K23TC

Wikipedia. "Nursing Home Administrator: Job Description and Career Info." Retrieved from https://study.com/articles/nursing-Home-Administrator_Job_Description_and_Info_for_Students_Considering_a_Career_in_Nursing_Home_Administration.html

Wikipedia. "Organization." Retrieved from businessdictionary.com/definition/organization.html

Wikipedia. "Organization: Meaning, Definition, Concepts and Characteristics." Retrieved from yourarticlelibrary.com/organization-meaning-definition-concepts-and-characteristics/53217

Wikipedia. "Holism x Reductionism." Retrieved from https://managementmania.com/en/holism-reductionism

Wikipedia. "Holistic Management." Retrieved from insideoutsidemgmt.com.au/holistic-management

Wikipedia. "The Difference a Holistic Business Approach Makes." Retrieved from sixsigmaonline/six-sigma-training-certification-information/the-difference-a-holistic-business-approach-makes

Wikipedia. "Stephen Convey Quotes>Quotable Quotes." Retrieved from https://www.goodreads.com/quotes/104483-i-am-not-a-product-of-my-circumstanes-i-am

Wikipedia. "The Importance of CNAs in Long Term Care." Retrieved from premiernursingacademy.org/blog/the-importance-of-cnas-in-long-term-care/

Wikipedia. "Medicine and Technology." Retrieved from www.health carebusinesstech.com/medical-technology/

Wikipedia. "Allan Savory." Retrieved from https://wikipedia.org/wiki/Allan-Savory

Wikipedia. "Why Holistic Management." Retrieved from holistic management.org/holistic-management/

Wikipedia. "What Are Holistic Approaches and Why Aew Companies Using Them?" Retrieved from beyo.global/thinking/what-are-holistic -approaches-and-why-are-companies-using-them

Appendix

CROSSWALK – OLD AND NEW FEDERAL NURSING HOME REGULATIONS
Department of Health Services / Division of Quality Assurance
P-01943 (08/2017)

Effective November 28, 2017, The Centers for Medicare and Medicaid Services (CMS) will re-organize and re-number the federal nursing home requirements found in Appendix PP. This publication matches the federal nursing home tags from Appendix PP in the November 2016 Mega Rule with the new tag numbers effective 11/28/17.

Old Tag	New Tag	Description
F150	F540	Definition of facility – SNF and NF
F151	F550	Right to exercise rights/free of reprisal
F152	F551	Rights exercised by representative
F153	F573	Right to access/purchase copies of record
F154	F552	Informed of health status, care and treatments
F154	F552	Right to be informed of changes to the plan of care
F155	F578	Right to refuse treatment and formulate advance directive
F155	F678	CPR given while EMTs are en route
F156	F574	Required notices and contact information
F156	F575	Information required to be posted
F156	F579	Oral and written information about how to apply for and use Medicare and Medicaid benefits
F156	F582	Information provided to Medicaid-eligible residents; notification of changes in coverage
F156	F572	Inform resident of rights and services and facility rules
F157	F580	Prompt consultation with physician following significant condition change
F158	F567	Right to manage own financial affairs
F159	F567	Facility management of personal funds
F159	F568	Accounting and record of each resident's personal funds
F159	F569	Notice of certain balances
F160	F569	Conveyance of personal funds after death/discharge
F161	F570	Surety bond
F162	F571	Limitation on charges to personal funds
F163	F555	Right to choose attending physician
F164	F583	Personal privacy and confidentiality of record
F164	F842	Information in medical record kept confidential and released only in specific situations
F165	F585	Right to voice grievances without reprisal
F166	F585	Right to prompt efforts to resolve grievances
F167	F577	Right to view survey results; readily accessible
F168	F577	Right to info from and contact with advocate agencies
F168	F586	Must not prohibit or discourage a resident from communicating with federal, state, local officials
F169	F566	Right to choose to perform or refuse to do services for the facility
F170	F576	Right to privacy – send/receive unopened mail
F171	F576	Right to communicate with individuals inside/out; right to send mail and have access to postage
F172	F563	Right to receive/deny visitors
F172	F564	Immediate access to resident
F173	F583	Allow ombudsmen to access record
F174	F576	Right to telephone access with privacy
F175	F559	Right to share room with spouse or roommate of choice
F176	F554	Resident allowed to self-administer drugs if deemed safe
F177	F560	Right to refuse certain transfers

Old Tag	New Tag	Description
F201	F622	Reasons for transfer/discharge of a resident
F202	F622	Documentation for transfer/discharge of a resident
F203	F623	Notice requirements for transfer/discharge
F204	F624	Preparation for safe/orderly transfer or discharge
F205	F625	Notice of bed-hold policy before/upon transfer
F206	F626	Policy to permit readmission beyond bed hold
F207	F621	Equal practices regardless of payment source
F208	F620	Prohibiting certain admission policies
F221	F604	Right to be free from physical restraints
F222	F605	Right to be free from chemical restraints
F223	F600	Right to be free from abuse and neglect
F223	F602	Right to be free from misappropriation and exploitation
F223	F603	Right to be free from involuntary seclusion
F224	F600	Must not use verbal/physical/sexual abuse, corporal punishment, or involuntary seclusion
F225	F606	Not employ/engage staff with adverse actions
F225	F609	Report allegations of abuse, neglect, misappropriation
F225	F610	Investigate allegations of abuse and neglect, misappropriation and prevent further occurrence
F226	F607	Develop/implement policies prohibiting abuse/neglect/misappropriation/exploitation
F226	F943	Abuse, neglect, and exploitation training
F240	F550	Care and environment promotes quality of life
F240	F550	Equal access to quality care
F241	F550	Dignity and respect of individuality
F242	F561	Self-determinations; right to make choices
F243	F565	Right to organize and participate in resident groups
F244	F565	Facility must consider views of resident or family group and act promptly on them
F245	F561	Right to participate in other activities
F246	F558	Reasonable accommodation of needs and preferences
F247	F559	Right to notice before room or roommate change
F248	F679	Activities meet interests/needs of each resident
F249	F680	Qualifications of activity professional
F250	F745	Provision of medically-related social services
F251	F850	Qualifications of social worker > 120 beds
F252	F584	Safe/clean/comfortable/homelike environment
F252	F557	Right to use personal possessions
F253	F584	Housekeeping and maintenance services to maintain sanitary, orderly, comfortable interior
F254	F584	Clean bed/bath linens in good condition
F256	F584	Adequate and comfortable lighting levels
F257	F584	Comfortable and safe temperature levels
F258	F584	Maintenance of comfortable sound levels
F271	F635	Must have physician orders for admission
F272	F636	Comprehensive assessments
F273	F636	Comprehensive assessment completed by 14 days after admission
F274	F637	Comprehensive assessment after significant change in condition
F275	F636	Comprehensive assessment at least every 12 months
F276	F638	Quarterly assessment at least every three months
F278	F641	Assessment accuracy/coordination/certified

Old Tag	New Tag	Description
F278	F642	Coordinate assessments with appropriate participation of health professionals
F279	F656	Develop comprehensive care plans
F279	F639	Maintain all assessments completed within the last 15 months
F280	F657	Comprehensive care plan developed within 7 days
F280	F553	Right to participate in planning and revision of care plan
F281	F658	Services provided meet professional standards
F282	F659	Services by qualified person in accordance with care plan
F283	F661	Items to be included in discharge summary
F284	F660	Must develop and implement a discharge planning process
F284	F661	When discharge is anticipated, facility must develop a post-discharge plan of care
F285	F644	Coordination of PASARR and assessments
F285	F645	PASARR screening requirements for MI and MR
F285	F646	MD/ID significant change notification
F286	F639	Maintain all assessments completed within the last 15 months
F287	F640	Encoding/transmitting resident assessment
F309	F675	Quality of life
F309	F684	Quality of care – promote highest practicable level of well-being
F309	F697	Pain management
F309	F744	Dementia care
F309	F698	Dialysis
F309	F684	End of life care
F310	F676	Activities of daily living do not diminish
F311	F676	Appropriate services to improve or maintain activities of daily living
F312	F677	ADL care provided for dependent residents
F313	F685	Assist resident in making appointment/transportation to/from vision and hearing appointments
F314	F686	Treatment/services to prevent/heal pressure injuries
F315	F690	No catheter; services to promote urinary continence
F317	F688	Resident does not experience reduction in range of motion, unless unavoidable
F318	F688	Increase/prevent decrease in range of motion
F319	F742	Appropriate treatment and services to those with psychosocial adjustment difficulty
F320	F743	No pattern of behavioral difficulties unless unavoidable
F322	F693	No feeding tubes unless necessary; restore oral eating; prevent complication of enteral feeding
F323	F689	Free of accident hazards/supervision and assistive devices to prevent accidents
F323	F700	Bedrails
F325	F692	Maintain nutritional status unless unavoidable
F327	F692	Sufficient fluid to maintain hydration status
F328	F687	Foot care
F328	F691	Colostomy, urostomy, or ileostomy care.
F328	F694	Parenteral fluids must be administered consistent with professional standards of practice
F328	F695	Respiratory care is provided in accordance with professional standards of practice
F328	F696	A resident with a prosthesis is provided care consistent with professional standards of practice
F329	F757	Drug regimen free of unnecessary drugs
F329	F758	Free of psychotropic drugs unless necessary; gradual dose reduction for those on psychotropic meds
F332	F759	Free of medication error rate of 5% or more
F333	F760	Facility is free of significant medication errors
F334	F883	Influenza and pneumococcal vaccinations

Old Tag	New Tag	Description
F353	F725	Adequate staffing to meet needs of residents
F353	F726	Competent nursing staff
F354	F727	RN 8 hours/day, 7 days/week; full-time DON
F355	F731	Waiver of 24-hour licensed nurse and RN coverage
F356	F732	Posted nurse staffing information
F360	F800	Provided diet meets needs of each resident
F361	F801	Sufficient/qualified staff to carry out functions of food service; qualified dietitian
F362	F802	Sufficient support personnel to carry out the function of food and nutrition service
F363	F803	Menus meet resident needs/prepared in advance and followed
F364	F804	Food maintains nutritive value; food/drink palatable, attractive, at safe and appetizing temp
F365	F805	Food in form to meet individual needs
F366	F806	Food accommodates resident allergies, intolerance, and preferences
F366	F806	Appealing options of similar nutritive value to those requesting a different meal choice
F366	F807	Provide drinks consistent with resident needs to maintain resident hydration
F367	F808	Therapeutic diet prescribed by physician
F368	F809	Meal frequency and snacks
F369	F810	Assistive devices/eating equipment and utensils
F371	F812	Store, prepare, distribute, and serve food under sanitary conditions
F371	F813	Have a policy for use and storage of food brought to residents by family and others
F372	F814	Dispose garbage and refuse properly
F373	F811	Feeding assistant – training and supervision; selection of residents
F373	F948	Training for feeding assistants
F385	F710	Resident's care supervised by a physician
F386	F711	Physician visits – review care; write and sign progress notes; sign and date new orders
F387	F712	Frequency of MD visits
F388	F712	Alternate visits by nurse practitioner, physician assistant or clinical nurse specialist
F389	F713	Physician for emergency care available 24 hours/day
F390	F714	Physician delegation of tasks to nurse practitioner, physician assistant, clinical nurse specialist
F390	F715	Physician delegation of tasks to dietitian/therapist
F406	F825	Provide/obtain specialized rehab services
F407	F826	Specialized rehab services ordered by MD and provided by qualified personnel
F411	F790	Routine/emergency dental services in SNFs
F412	F791	Routine/emergency dental services in NFs
F425	F755	Pharmaceutical services ensure accurate acquiring, receiving, administering
F428	F756	Drug regimen review, report and act on irregularities
F428	F758	Definition of a psychotropic drug
F431	F761	Labeling and storing of drugs and biologicals
F431	F755	Must employ services of a licensed pharmacist
F441	F880	Infection control program to prevent spread of infection
F454	F905	Physical environment
F455	K-tag	Emergency power
F455	F907	Space and equipment in dining/health services/recreation/program areas
F456	F908	Essential equipment maintained in safe operating condition
F456	F910	Bedrooms designed/equipped for adequate nursing care, comfort, and privacy
F457	F911	Bedrooms must accommodate no more than four residents
F458	F912	Bedrooms measure at least 80 square feet/resident

Old Tag	New Tag	Description
F459	F913	Bedroom has direct access to an exit corridor
F460	F914	Bedrooms assure full visual privacy
F461	F584	Each bedroom has private closet space
F461	F700	Follow manufacturer's recommendations for installing and maintaining bed rails
F461	F909	Regular inspection of bedframes, mattress, and bed rails
F461	F915	Bedroom has at least one window
F461	F916	Bedroom at or above grade level
F461	F916	Resident room bed/mattress/furniture/closet
F462	F918	Bedroom located with or near toilet and bathing facilities
F463	F919	Resident call system
F464	F920	Requirements for dining and activity rooms
F465	F921	Safe/functional/sanitary/comfortable environment
F466	F922	Procedures to ensure water availability
F467	F923	Window or mechanical ventilation
F468	F924	Corridors have firmly secured handrails
F469	F925	Maintains effective pest control program
F496	F729	Nurse aide registry verification/retraining
F490	F835	Administration
F491	F836	Facility is licensed by State
F492	F836	In compliance with all applicable federal, state, and local laws
F493	F837	Governing body
F494	F728	Must not use nurse aide for > 4 months unless competent and has completed nurse aide trng
F495	F728	Must not use nurse aide who has worked < 4 months unless in a nurse aide training program
F496	F729	Nurse aide registry verification, retraining
F497	F730	Nurse aide performance review every 12 months
F498	F726	Proficiency of nurse aides
F498	F947	In-service training of nurse aides
F499	F839	Staff qualifications
F500	F840	Outside professional resources – arrangement/agreement
F501	F841	Responsibilities of Medical Director
F502	F770	Must provide or obtain laboratory services
F502	F771	Must provide or obtain laboratory services (blood bank and transfusion)
F503	F770	Must meet requirements for laboratory services if provided onsite
F503	F771	Must meet requirements for blood bank and transfusion services if provided onsite
F503	No tag	Referring laboratory must be certified in appropriate specialties and subspecialties
F503	F772	Must have an agreement for laboratory services if not provided onsite
F504	F773	Lab services only when ordered by MD
F505	F773	Promptly notify MD of lab results that fall outside clinical reference range
F506	F774	Assist resident in making transportation arrangements to source of service
F507	F775	File laboratory results in clinical record
F508	F776	Provide or obtain radiology and other diagnostic services
F509	F776	Diagnostic services meet standards for such services
F510	F777	Obtain radiology/diagnostic services only when ordered
F511	F777	Promptly notify MD of diagnostic results that fall outside of clinical reference ranges
F512	F778	Assist resident in making transportation arrangements to radiology
F513	F779	File radiology/diagnostic results in clinical record

Old Tag	New Tag	Description
F514	F842	Documentation in accordance with professional standards of quality
F515	F842	Retention of records
F516	F842	Must not release information that is resident identifiable
F516	F842	Safeguard medical record against loss
F517	F838	Detailed plans and procedures to meet potential emergencies and disasters
F518	No tag	Train all employees in emergency procedures
F519	F843	Transfer agreement
F520	F865	QAPI program/plan. disclosure/good faith attempts
F520	F866	QAPI/QAA data collection and monitoring
F520	F867	QAPI/QAA improvement activities
F520	F868	QAA committee
F522	F844	Disclosure of ownership
F523	F845	Facility closure – administrator responsibilities
F524	F846	Policies and procedures in place in event of facility closure
F525	No tag	Binding arbitration agreements
F526	F849	Hospice services
F527	F851	Mandatory submission of staffing information based on payroll

Administrators' Daily Quiz

In a holistic nursing home management, which of the following objectives is most important to you and organization?

A. Maintain the highest resident quality care
B. Maintain the highest daily census
C. Maintain the highest staffing and staff motivational levels
D. A and B
E. A and C
F. B and C
G. None of the above
H. All of the above

Index

www.ingramcontent.com/pod-product-compliance
Lightning Source LLC
Chambersburg PA
CBHW021351210526
45463CB00001B/67